The Gaying of America
&
The ~~Judgement~~ Love of God

M.A.R.

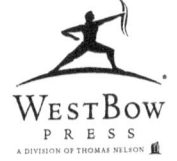

WESTBOW
PRESS
A DIVISION OF THOMAS NELSON

Scripture taken from the King James Version of the Bible.

Author Credits: compiler of "God's Book of Prayers" & "The Lord's Prayers"

WestBow Press books may be ordered through booksellers or by contacting:

WestBow Press
A Division of Thomas Nelson
1663 Liberty Drive
Bloomington, IN 47403
www.westbowpress.com
1 (866) 928-1240

ISBN: 978-1-4908-2087-3 (sc)
ISBN: 978-1-4908-2088-0 (e)

Library of Congress Control Number: 2013923355

Printed in the United States of America.
WestBow Press rev. date: 12/30/2013

Contents

Dedication vii

Foreword..ix

Introduction..xiii

1. What God Is All About...1

2. The Greatest of These Is Love 13

3. What God Has to Say about Homosexuality........25

4. Sodom and Gomorrah: A Revised History...........39

5. The Prenatal Holocaust.......................................47

6. The Decay and Fall of the American Empire........53

7. What Should We Then Do?...................................77

8. Out of the Closet and into the Light! 87

Appendix 101

Chapter Notes...125

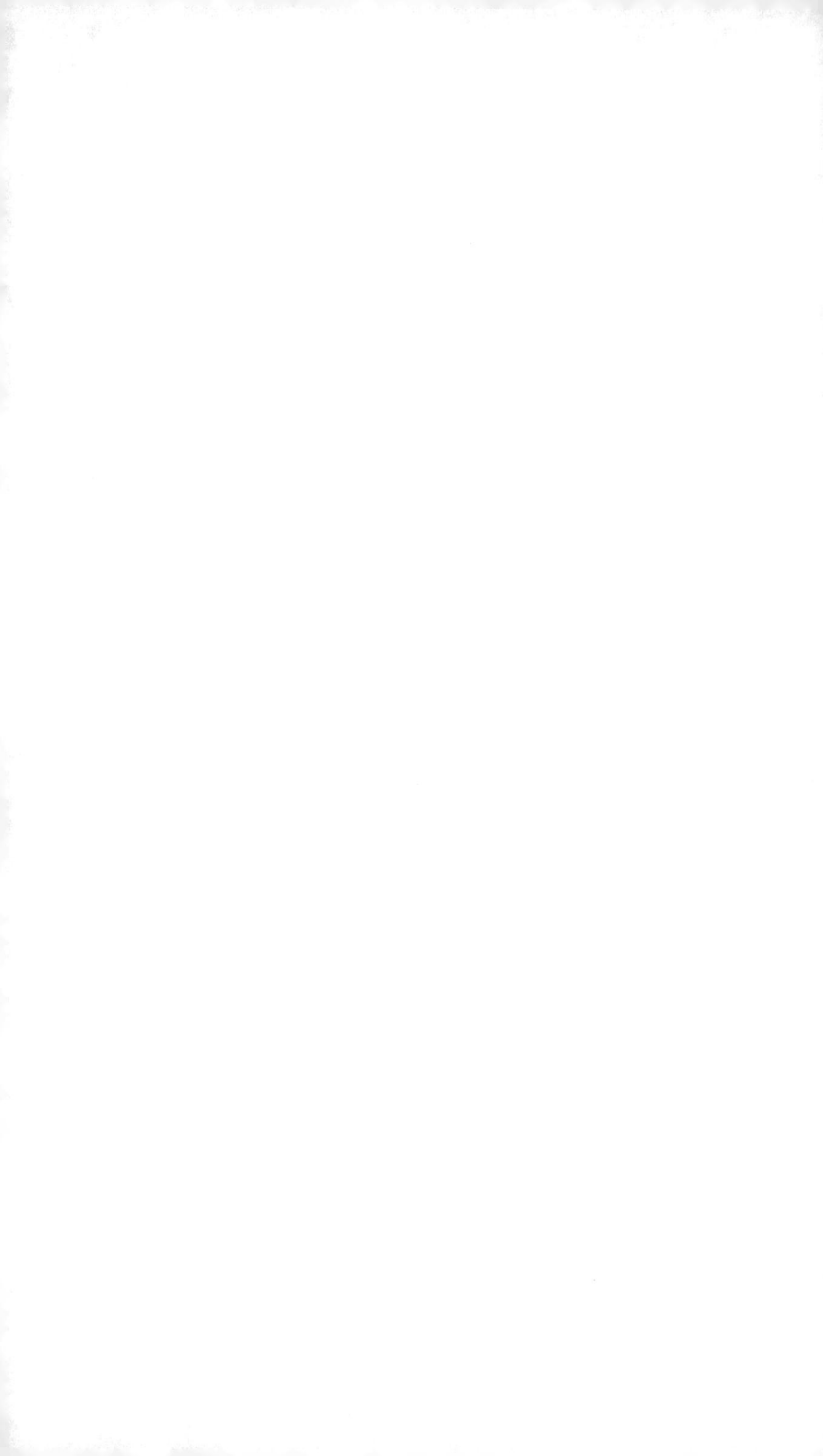

Dedication

In honor of the church congregation of
Victory in Jesus in Okinawa, Japan
during the 1980s and 1990s.
The founders and leaders,
David Drueding and Mary Drueding Derringer,
were the first to teach us about the kingdom of God.
That knowledge has forever transformed
the lives of hundreds of us.

Foreword

It is my distinct honor to have been asked to write the foreword to *The Gaying of America and The Love of God* written by M. A. R. I have known the author of this book for many years. I know him to be a conscientious and keen student of the Word of God. This fact is well illustrated by his first work, *God's Book of Prayers,* which can be found at www.GodsBookOfPrayers.com.

Centuries ago, the wise Solomon said, "of making many books there is no end" (Ecclesiastes 12:12). The apostle John said of Jesus, "And there are also many other things which Jesus did, the which, if they should be written every one, I suppose that even the world itself could not contain the books that should be written. Amen" (John 21:25). Solomon himself wrote 3,000 proverbs and 1,005 songs per 1 Kings 4:32. Thus, the task becomes distinguishing between the ordinary and the extraordinary.

The author of this work took it upon himself to write about a very difficult, sensitive, and divisive subject. Although others have written about this subject, M. A. R. has written with sensitivity and compassion toward those who are wrapped up in the trappings of the sin of homosexuality. He discusses the matter with love and without compromising God's Word. This is no ordinary work.

M. A. R.'s writing exemplifies the principles espoused in St. John 3:16, 17: "For God so loved the world, that He gave His only begotten Son, that whosoever believes in Him, should not perish, but have everlasting life. For God sent not His Son into the world to condemn the world; but that the world through Him might be saved." The true Christian believer's primary responsibility in this matter is deduced from Scripture and wonderfully explained.

The book also includes a very touching testimony from someone who was caught in the trap of his destructive behavior and lifestyle before being delivered from his dilemma.

I wholeheartedly recommend this book to anyone who is in the throes of this sort of behavior and wants to be delivered from it. Likewise, I sincerely recommend *The Gaying of America and The Love of God* for all who want to understand God's view of homosexuality. Especially important are the portions that deal with the unconditional love of God underlying—yet not undoing—His judgment.

This final word is for proponents and opponents of same-sex marriage, believers and unbelievers in God: if you begin to read this work, please continue to the end. The book contains sobering advice for people on each side of this issue. Do not get bogged down by passages that offend you; after all, the very next page may include an idea that speaks to you meaningfully or provides some interesting insight or important piece of information on the subject.

Rev. Guadalupe Rodriguez
VA chaplain, retired
MDiv

Introduction

Over the past several years, we have seen a rising societal acceptance of relationships that deviate from one man and one woman. Given the fact that the Supreme Court of the United States recently heard arguments about same-sex marriage, it seems inevitable that they will one day approve that arrangement. If they do not, individual states are already beginning to allow same-sex marriage one by one. Seeking to end same-sex marriage is a hard argument to win in human terms. After all, it appears to be an equality issue. Indeed, *marriage equality* is the phrase being used by gay marriage advocates.

What should prevent someone from marrying whichever sex they choose? *Equal rights* has long been America's mantra, since the American Civil War days. True Christians were against slavery because God made all people, and nobody has the right to decide one race is better than the others. In the twentieth century, America saw the advent of civil rights, child rights, worker rights, disabled rights, and many other rights. Although it has been said that God helps those who help themselves, I believe that God is more on the side of those who *cannot* help themselves. God and His true people were on the side of the maltreated in all of the aforementioned movements.

So now that the twenty-first century has arrived and is in full swing, why wouldn't God and God's people be on the side of this newest group of people being discriminated against? There is one simple truth that separates today's gay rights movement from all of the previous movements in America, and it is clearly stated in the Bible. The Bible is God's own words; He dictated to human writers what came from His heart and mind.

Whichever side one finds oneself on when contemplating this issue, we all must marvel at how quickly the gay rights movement gained traction over the past several years. I am not entirely shocked by the emergence of the homosexual movement in the world today, just as I am not shocked by the countless natural catastrophes and the increase in violence in many parts of the world as of late—events foretold in the Bible.

Many expected such events to happen as time went on, but I did not expect to see them all happen in my lifetime.

This movement may not be the very end; however, if not, it will bring us closer to the end. After all, mankind is taking another large step away from God's ways.

Does God hate the homosexual person? No. Does God hate the thief? No. Does God hate the liar? No. I echo all those *nos,* as do all true children of God. This book is not about hatred or darkness; it is about showing God's love, light, and life to all communities. By the same token, this book is not a compromised reading of the Bible. After all, what right do I have to compromise God's Word? God's Word is sacred, and for me to modify it in any manner would be blasphemous. Instead, I want to show what God has to say about this sensitive topic.

We are supposed to treat everyone with dignity and respect. As people in society, we should not discriminate against anyone. God did not call us to discriminate; instead, He called us to love. As we can plainly see in the Bible, there are more references to God's love than to sexual sins, including homosexuality. The church should be leading the way in reaching out to all sinners, including the LGBT (lesbian, gay, bisexual, transgender) community.

Love will cover a multitude of sins. Peter, the apostle, informs us of that fact. James, the apostle, instructs us to notify sinners of the error of their ways in order to save their soul from death. By so doing, we will have covered over and helped cleanse a multitude of sins.[1] We need to know about God's holy standards, and we can only be truly aware of them through what we read in the Holy Scripture, the Bible.

Many in the Christian community willingly inform others of sin, but far fewer convey genuine love toward those same sinners (even though we are, or were, in the same boat). If we are believers, followers of God in Jesus Christ, we know of and have experienced God's mercy and grace. That concept is what this book is all about: showing God's loving Law, extending God's love through His mercy and grace, and growing God's kingdom by as many as will come to God. This notion is described in Isaiah, chapter 26: "Open you the gates, that the righteous nation which keeps the truth may enter in. You will keep him in perfect peace, whose mind is stayed on You: because he trusts in You. The way of the just is uprightness: Thou, most upright, dost weigh the path of the just."[2] The multitude of God's mercies far outweigh the multitude of our sins.[3]

Unfortunately, though, the sin of openly accepted homosexuality—with the help of legally authorized same-sex marriage—may be the last in the long line of sins against God and mankind. People are beginning to shake their fists at God in a very real, public, and haughty manner. In essence, some are proclaiming to the Lord God, Creator of the universe, that they no longer respect Him or even acknowledge His existence.

The same God who created the world authored the universal laws that societies live by, including laws that prohibit homosexuality. We cannot pick and choose which of His universal laws we will live by. God's view will be explored in this writing, in addition to the very heart of God. I will also explore some possible reasons for these commandments. Does God hate sin, and specifically, the sin of homosexuality? Scripture is very clear on this.

Sadly the United States of America is drifting further and further away from the God who created us. Meanwhile, God continues to love us deeply. Luke 15:20 provides an account of God running to meet and love one of His sinner children. America continues running away from God, even though God continues to love America. We run toward riches, pleasure, and the opposite of God's eternal laws. Still, He loves us.

Deliverance is available for any person who turns to God and confronts the error of his or her ways. Many people have been delivered from their errant lifestyle by the grace, love, and help of God. God, the very definition of love, is sincerely concerned about all trapped in homosexual lifestyles and wants His people to emulate His love and concern for His most prized creation: humanity.

I have been a believer in Jesus for thirty-two years, and I was raised as a conservative in a sometimes critical and judgmental environment. But this work has transformed my thinking on this issue. Before, I leaned toward hellfire preaching when it came to such behavior, but God did a wonderful work on me as I researched for and wrote this book. In time, I learned to better understand God's love of us all. May God inspire similar feeling in those already on my side of the aisle; may God incite an awakening of the spirit in those who do not believe.

1

What God Is All About

John, the apostle, tells us some absolutes regarding God. In 1 John 4:8b, he says that "God is love" and at 1 John 1:5b, he says that "God is light" …. There is no darkness, nor hatred, nor condemnation in Him. Based on that statement, I know that God does *not* hate the gay community; in fact, God loves gay people. What I mentioned in the introduction is worth reviewing; I want everyone to have a better sense of what is in my own heart.

God does *not* hate the gay person.

God did not send His Son into the world to condemn the world; He sent His Son to save the world.[1] Luke relates the incident of Jesus rebuking two of His disciples, James and John, for wanting to command fire from heaven and annihilate some people who would not treat Jesus properly. Jesus stated, "You know not what manner of spirit you are of for the Son of Man is not come to destroy people's lives, but to save them."[2] Neither did God call us, any of His children, out of the world to condemn the rest of humanity. Instead we should love others and tell them about God's love for them.

The two most definitive characteristics of God are His love and His holiness. His holiness is His nature, which cannot be changed; God's love is how He is because He chooses to be that way. How much did God choose to love humanity? His signature act, of course, can be found in the well-known John 3:16 passage. Jesus' nature is holiness; He has no wickedness. But Jesus chose to love us in our wickedness and acted on that love by leaving His heavenly kingdom to come to earth and live among us.

Jesus came not only to live, but also to die for us, to provide the way back to God that we had lost. So God is holy, and He chooses to be loving. Jesus chose to love us by coming down to earth and giving His life for us. We were created a certain way, with certain characteristics that make us who we are as individuals and as a society. God designed us a certain way and it brings Him great joy when we live according to His ways; however, it must break His heart when we break His plan.

As God chooses to love, so must we choose to love. God created us so that we could have a relationship with Him and meet with Him, but because we cannot truly approach Him in His holiness, God extends mercy and grace to us. We are to operate in His love – via mercy and grace – extending this same behavior to all, including homosexuals. In Exodus 25:21, God reveals His holiness in His law and His love in His mercy (through the ark of the covenant and its associated components).

"And you shall put the mercy seat above upon the ark; and in the ark you shall put the Testimony that I shall give you. And there I will meet with you."[3] This is a wonderful indication of how God continues to deal with the human race. After God had given the testimony (Ten Commandments) to the people, He went on to tell Moses that he needed to build a proper house for God, a house to hold the ark of the covenant. The ark of the covenant is surely the most treasured possession of the Jewish nation.

The ark is so precious because, through it, God stated that He would meet with the people. Interestingly, God did not say, that such a meeting was contingent upon the Ten Commandments inside the ark; instead, he explained that His mercy would be the enabling factor.[4] This ark remains symbolic of how God deals with everyone, even today. Inside the ark is the law of God, which expresses the holiness of God. The mercy seat covers the ark, and it indicates God's love.

God said that He would meet with us at the covering (the lid) of the ark, otherwise known as the mercy seat. It is impossible for us to approach what is inside the ark without God reaching out to us at the mercy seat. God shows His love by extending mercy and grace to us. He reveals His holiness to us via His love. God asks us to live by His love so that we can reach holiness.

Jesus came into this world to save the world, not to condemn anyone.[5]

The topic of this book is a small portion of God's law that informs us what sort of behavior is proper in terms of this area of human sexuality. God's other defining characteristic, love, teaches us how to deal, lovingly, with those who violate this portion of His law. Remember: Jesus came into this world to save the world, not to condemn anyone.[5]

Love and Life

Of course, John's most famous quote is found in John 3:16: "For God so loved the world, that He gave His only begotten Son, that whosoever believeth in Him should not perish, but have everlasting life." It is the very next verse that informs us that "God sent not His Son in the world to condemn the world; but that the world through Him might be saved."[6] Jesus came into the world to save us, not to destroy us. It is the enemy of our souls, Satan, who came to destroy us. God stated that anyone could come to Jesus to avoid death.

The result of not dying is that we have everlasting life. When we come to God as we are, God will rescue us from death and offer us abundant life.[7] The new life He gives us applies not only to our future afterlives, but also to our current, earthly lives. We cannot, however, continue living our life on earth from that point on, the point at which God rescues us, in the same manner as we lived in the past. A change in soul status necessitates a change in living status. Jesus gave His life so that we could and would walk away from sin. He expects us to conform ourselves to His Word.

We cannot, from the point at which God rescues us, continue living our life on earth in the same manner as we lived in the past.

Luke 1:74–75 tells us that the Lord enables us to serve Him during the entirety of our rescued lives. Added to that, we are enabled to serve Him in *holiness* and *righteousness* throughout our new life. God be blessed, who not only rescued us from death, but also strengthened us so we could live in the manner that He requires! Paul, the apostle, wrote that he labored struggling with all of God's energy that was working so powerfully in him.[8] It is all of God's energy and not our own!

What was it that transformed John from one who condemned – a "son of thunder" (remember, he was one of the brothers who wanted to command fire from heaven in order to annihilate people) – into one known as the apostle of love? His miraculous transformation was brought about by his relationship with Jesus. When we truly meet the God of the universe, we will never be the same.

When Jesus touches us, He enables us to change ourselves and stop living lives of sin. We all have some sin to overcome, and overcome we must if we are to be close with God. God will radically and entirely change us if we allow Him to, but we must willingly forsake our sinful ways and follow God's Word in every area of our life.

God is able to change us into who He wants us to be, even though we may have lived in the dark for years. No longer will we want to live in shadow; rather, we will want to live as God wants us to live. Like a photographer, God can take the negatives in our lives and transform them into fully developed positives. We will be able to bless God and remember all of His many and varied benefits in our lives.[9]

God loves us all tremendously. He created us so we could love Him, and so that He could shed His love on us. God also wants us to live according to the ways that He has shown us: His correct ways. He will not reject anyone who turns to Him. However, we must turn to God and reject (or die to) our erroneous ways. Titus 2:11 states that, "the grace of God that brings salvation appears to all of us."

God can take the negatives in your life and transform them into fully developed positives.

We should be a mirror reflecting the image of Christ; so that when others look at us, they should see Jesus. The Greek word for *grace* is *charis,* which literally means *the divine influence upon the heart, and its reflection in the life.*[10] As the Lord influences our hearts, we must reflect that divine influence in our own lives. Even though the popular acronym G.R.A.C.E. (God's Riches at Christ's Expense) is true, many have not experienced the grace of God truly because it is not reflected in their lives.

Much of the Lord's influence on us comes from His Holy Word. The Bible is necessary for our lives because it comes directly from God and empowers us to live the life that we should live. The Scripture is food for our spirit and soul just as ordinary food is nourishment for our physical bodies. The Scripture breathes life into our spirits just as God breathed life into Adam.

Physically, the Lord breathed into man's nostrils the breath of life and man became a living soul.[11] Spiritually, the Bible is the divine breath of God into our spirits. It gives us His life so that the person of God is thoroughly furnished for all good works.[12] God expects us to conform ourselves to His Holy Word, to change based on our new understandings and to perform good works that He destined us to perform. A popular portion of Scripture that speaks about the grace of God and the ability of faith in God to bring about salvation also tells us that He created us and predestined us to do good deeds.

"For by grace are ye saved through faith; and that not of yourselves: it is the gift of God: not of works, lest any man should boast. For we are His workmanship, created in Christ Jesus unto good works, which God hath before ordained that we should walk in them."[13] We must review God's Word carefully because, as Jesus told us, in Scripture is eternal life.[14]

God's Will and Testament

God declares that He reaches out to us every day in every way because, often, we live in a way that is not good. What is that *not good* way? Isaiah 65:2 states that we are not doing well when we live "after our own thoughts." We must shun our own thoughts about how we should live. As mandated, we must die to ourselves and our ways in favor of God's ways.

God's ways of living are found in His Holy Word. The Bible is explicit and replete with admonitions to live according to God's will. To initiate a person's last will and testament, it is necessary for that person to be dead. In this case, for God's will to be initiated in our lives, we must die. The will of God requires the death of someone. Actually, God's will requires two deaths. Jesus already gave His life, and now it is our responsibility to die. To implement

God's will in your life, you must give your life. God will not release His will in your life until you relinquish your own will. In order to understand this better, it is helpful to look at the first instance of the death of a person.

Genesis, chapter 3, informs us of the circumstances and the actual act that led to death in the human race. Mankind was tempted by Satan to do that which God commanded mankind not to do. The enemy showed Eve (and Adam, who was with her) that the forbidden tree was good for food, was pleasing to the eye, and could make one wise. Satan declared that they would not die if they ate the fruit.

Of course, that act led to the spiritual and physical death of Adam, Eve, and the entire human race. Death was never a part of the will of God for humanity, but occurred due to their disobedience. If Adam and Eve would have been obedient and submitted to the will of God, in other words, if they would have died to their own will, or desires, it would have ended better for them.

**The death of someone is required
for a will to take effect.
God's will in your life requires
the death of your own will.**

We would all be lost forever had it not been for the "last Adam" who came from heaven.[15] In 1 John 2:15–17, John expects us to "love not the world, neither the things that are in the world … For all that is in the world, the lust of the flesh, and the lust of the eyes, and the pride of life, is not of the Father, but is of the world. And the world passes away, and the lust thereof: but he that does the will of God abides forever." Notice that the three categories of "all that is in the world" are the very areas that doomed Adam and Eve. They died because they fell to "the lust of the flesh, and the lust of the eyes, and the pride of life." The first Adam did not overcome the temptations of this world, but Jesus, the last Adam, did!

Both Matthew 4:1–11 and Luke 4:1–13 speak of the temptation of Jesus: the same Satan came to Jesus and presented the very same arguments to Jesus that he had proposed to Adam and Eve. Satan tempted Jesus with what John described and what Adam and Eve experienced, namely physical satisfaction, material things, and pride of life.

And how did Jesus refute the enemy? First of all, Jesus prepared for the battle that the Devil was going to initiate against him. The Scripture tells us that, just after Jesus was baptized, He separated Himself from others by going into the wilderness—2 Corinthians 6:17 states, "Wherefore come out from among them, and be ye separate, saith the Lord." That separation may refer to a spiritual event and not necessarily a physical event.

Jesus fasted for forty days and forty nights in the wilderness. After fasting for that long, Jesus was hungry. And that is when Satan began to tempt him. Every time Satan presented a temptation to Jesus, Jesus refuted him with words from the Scripture. Proper knowledge and application of the Scripture will ensure God's will and life in our lives. The greatest command we can apply in our lives is to love, and the greatest thing God offers us is love.

See the appendix for a continued discussion of what God is all about and a list of the times God stated, "I am." (The list is provided in an effort to show God's sovereignty and His stance toward mankind.) Following that list are the instances in the Bible when mankind stated the same phrase. I suspect you will see a distinct difference (and some similarities) between God's words and mankind's words.

2

The Greatest of These Is Love

We should seek to exhibit God's life in ourselves, especially as we interact with other people. 1 Corinthians 13:13 states, "And now abides faith, hope, love, these three; but the greatest of these is love." God does not have or need faith or hope. He does not need to believe in what He has done, is doing, or will do. God does not need to hope that the future will turn out in a certain way; He can effortlessly accomplish it or allow it to be accomplished. He does, however, experience love. In fact, God is love.

Of the greatest of the graces, the one that we have in common with Him is love. One might say that this is the common blood that flows between us. One can have faith without love and hope without love; but love believes in, trusts, and has hope in all things.[1] One's faith can fail; Jesus prayed that Peter's faith would not fail.[2]

We know that our hope can fail us, but the Scripture instructs us that love will never fail.[3] Faith and hope, in fact, will one day pass away. Conversely, love will always remain. After all, we will not need faith or hope in heaven because we will already have reached the apex of our hopes. In the glories of heaven, however, love will be ubiquitous.

God has many titles, including the following: Jehovah Jireh (provider), Jehovah Rohi (shepherd), Jehovah Rophe (healer), Jehovah Shalom (peace), Jehovah Shammah (the Lord is present), Jehovah Tsidkenu (righteousness), Jehovah Tsur (Rock), Savior, Counselor, Redeemer, Father, and Son of God. We have something in common with all these traits, at least on the lower end of the spectrum. We are powerful, yet we are not all-powerful beings; we are knowledgeable, yet we are not all-knowing beings; we can be present in one place, but we cannot be in all places at once. To some extent, we are able to heal, provide peace, and act in a righteous manner. But as far as love is concerned, God wants us to be equal with Him!

We can see love in the trinity: "God is love" and "God commended [exhibited] His love for us in that while we were yet sinners, Christ died for us."[4] God, the Father, didn't wait for us to stop sinning before He started loving us. Jesus didn't wait for us to love Him before He gave His life for us.

What about the Holy Spirit? We have the fruit of the Spirit listed in Galatians 5:22, 23. The first fruit listed is love. On packaged foods, the first ingredient mentioned on the label is typically the most prevalent one. Likewise, love is the first fruit—it is predominant with the Spirit, just as it should be with us.

The first fruit of the Spirit is love.

After recording the famous John 3:16, John recorded a second John 3:16. In the latter version, John repeats the previous words of God's love for the world, but he adds a word about our responsibility to apply that knowledge. In his first epistle, 1 John 3:16, the apostle states, "Hereby perceive we the love of God, because He [Jesus] laid down His life for us: and we ought to lay down our lives for the brethren." God calls us to reciprocate His love for the world by laying down our own lives for others. (See the following to learn the extent to which Jesus laid down His life for all of us.)

According to the Bible (see Philippians 2:1–8), we ought to be humble. Follow Jesus' example of humility in His descent from heaven:

Jesus, Son of God,
  King of Kings,
    Was in heaven above all.
      He lowered himself below the angels,
        Came down to earth,
          Became a man (but not a high man—not
          royalty or even middle class).
            He became a lowly man, a servant.
              He was born in a state lower than servants,
              among the animals.
                He was born in an animal's manger, not
                in a hospital or a house.
                  He lived as a poor man, even though He
                  is God;
                    He was rejected by man, His own
                    creation.
                      He was tortured before death:
                      He did not suffer an ordinary
                      death, he died on a cross,
                        Went below the earth (into the
                        grave),
                          Went further below the grave,

all the way to hell.
He suffered at the hands of
Satan in hell for you and me!

**Our Lord went from the *highest* position to the *lowest!*
Thus, do not complain about whatever it is that you
are dealing with. Be humble. If you need an example,
you only need to look to Jesus.**

A husband should love and care for his wife, and a
wife should honor and support her husband. Why is it
important to think of others before oneself, as mentioned
in Philippians 2:4? Out of the myriad obvious reasons,
I will look at a selfish reason. Much of the time, we look
out for our own interests and ways of looking good in
any given situation. In a sense, we want to make ourselves
larger than others. If we do things to help or promote our
own being, we may succeed and grow individually, but if
we do things to help or promote others, we will become
even bigger. How?

When I do things for myself only, the benefits are limited
to me. They will remain within my own skin, my own
being. I can only grow by one, as it were. When I do
things for another person, I can grow within that other
person. Thus, I can grow not just within myself for that

act, but also within that other person (and within some of their future acts). That growth is multiplied when the person I helped helps another, and so on. I then move on to the next person, and the effect becomes exponential. God has good reason to instruct us to help one another: by helping others, we help ourselves.

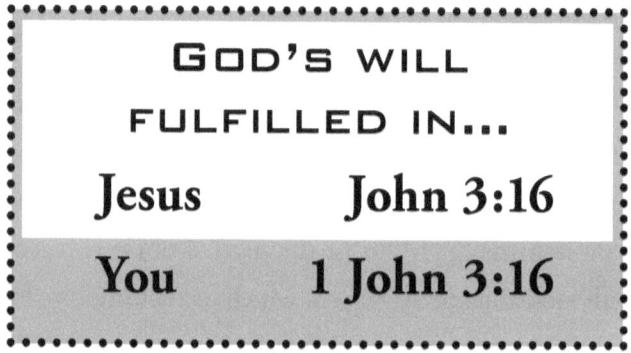

God transformed John's life: he went from a condemner, a "son of thunder," to the apostle of love! Early on, after he met Jesus, John wanted to destroy others; but in the end, he directed us to lay down our lives for others as Jesus did.[5] Our wills only last a lifetime, but those "that do the will of God abide forever." In order to live forever, we must die to ourselves to put into effect the will of God. Notice that the same terminology involving eternal life in John 3:16 is also found in 1 John 2:17.

John went from being a condemner, a "son of thunder," to being the apostle of love.

"And the world passes away, and the lust thereof: but he that does the will of God abides forever" (1 John 2:17). We must believe, which indicates a change of mind *and* a change of life, and we must do the will of God. What is God's will for us, and what does all this have to do with homosexuality and same-sex marrige?

The Will of God and Homosexuality

Many references to God's will can be found in Scripture, and none more famous than the Sermon on the Mount. Toward the end of that incredible speech, Jesus stressed that only those who do the will of God will enter heaven.[6] A similar mention is found in the first epistle to the Thessalonians in the third verse of chapter 4, wherein we learn that one major component of God's will is to be holy and abstain from sexual immorality.

Though God loves us infinitely, He will punish us for sexual immorality, as noted in the sixth verse of

19

1 Thessalonians chapter 4. Meanwhile in one Old Testament verse, we can see both the love of God and the judgment of God: Numbers 14:18 reads, "The Lord is longsuffering, and of great mercy [and love], forgiving iniquity and transgression, and by no means clearing the guilty."

Because God created this world, His rules apply to it. He is not judging us based upon rules applied after the fact. God told us clearly, in His own words, what we must do. Those words that were spoken before any one of us were around will judge us, and we can read them at any point in time.[7] To many people, this idea of God's love and judgment seems irreconcilable, even oxymoronic. After all, some say that a God of love couldn't judge anyone. How could a God of justice love? Those who struggle with this also find other apparent discrepancies with many of God's actions and words in the Bible.

For example, in both Matthew 27:44 and Mark 15:32, we are told that the two thieves who were crucified with Jesus mocked Jesus, as did many others. But in Luke 23:29–43, Scripture dictates that only one of the thieves crucified with Jesus mocked Him. Luke tells us that the other thief sided with Jesus and uttered the famous phrase, "Lord, remember me when Thou comest into Thy kingdom."

How do we reconcile these accounts? Were the Gospel writers mistaken? Or did one of them exaggerate the issue, thus lying? Well, no. There is a simple explanation which easily reconciles all the accounts, making every Word of God true. You see, both thieves on the crucifixion hill with Jesus, initially ridiculed and mocked Jesus. Then, after realizing his hollow words, the repentant thief stopped criticizing Jesus and began to rebuke his fellow thief. Thus, all accounts in the Gospel are true, even if they seem contradictory.

Many years ago, I wrestled with God's account of the creation of the world and what science was telling me. After all, how could the earth appear to be billions of years old when the Bible, via clear birth and death records, indicates that the earth is only thousands of years old? What about the dinosaurs? I wanted to believe scientists *and* the Bible, but I seemed to be facing an irreconcilable discrepancy. As I prayed and wrestled with this dilemma, the Lord revealed to me the truth inherent in both accounts.

In a single statement, God showed me that He created the earth with age built into it. In other words, the idea that the earth is billions of years old is true because God made it that way. Suppose a scientist had been on the scene the day after Adam was created and asked how old Adam was. The scientist would have studied Adam and reached the conclusion that Adam was perhaps twenty-five or thirty years old. In truth, though, Adam was only one day old because God had just created him the day before. What about a large tree that God had just made the day before? God created the tree with rings already built into it; otherwise, it would not have been a true tree. The tree that God made one day prior seemed to be dozens of years old.

The Lord further revealed to me that, though it seemed like the dinosaurs had roamed the earth, the earth was created with dinosaur bones imbedded into it. The Lord created the earth with oil and all other natural resources built into it. These resources, skeletons, artifacts, and other things did not take millions of years to develop—they were part of the earth that God had created just one day earlier.

The whole issue was cleared up from that point forward for me, and since then, I have believed in the advice offered by D. Elton Trueblood: "Faith is not evidence without proof, but trust without reservation."[8] Love and judgment are two characteristics of a righteous God. I have decided to trust God and His Word no matter which facts are presented to me. According to the eleventh chapter of Hebrews, that kind of faith is what the ancients were commended for.[9] We know faith is real because we can see it in creation, sense it in our conscience, and experience it in Christ.[10]

Even a gay person can come to Jesus just as he or she is.

God's acceptance of us is not a matter of *who* we are because God made us all. In fact, God even came to earth to live and die for all of us. God's acceptance of us is solely based upon His love for us. The door to heaven is open to all who accept God's death, burial, and resurrection; however, only those who live in the truth will enter heaven. Only those who live properly after accepting Jesus will enter heaven.[11]

Even a gay person can come to Christ Jesus just as he or she is. The message of Isaiah 1:18 applies here: "Come now, and let us reason together, says the Lord: though yours sins be as scarlet, they shall be as white as snow; though they be red like crimson, they shall be as wool." Thereafter a gay person must die to his or her own desires and live for God's, just as each and every one of us must die to our sins. Homosexuality is a sin, just as stealing and lying are sins, but homosexuality has a special connotation. As I will explain, the Bible has several things to say about the sin of homosexuality, both explicitly and implicitly.

3

What God Has to Say about Homosexuality

The Bible speaks clearly regarding how God feels about homosexuality. Leviticus 20:13 states, "If a man also lie with mankind, as he lies with a woman, both of them have committed an abomination." And Leviticus 18:22 indicates the same. In the New Testament, Paul informs us that homosexuals, among other unrighteous people, will not inherit the kingdom of God.[1] Paul goes on to state that some people were homosexual before they were washed and made holy. Those people were given the understanding that they could no longer continue living in that abominable way.[2]

> **If a man also lie with mankind, as he lies with a woman, both of them have committed an abomination. —Leviticus 20:13**

Some say that there is nothing wrong with choosing any marriage partner. However, those people often qualify that statement by saying that the choice must be within the parameters of the law. For instance, one cannot choose a child to be his or her spouse because man's law prohibits children from entering into marriage. Believers of God and His Word do not disagree with these words, but God's people will always choose God's laws over man's laws. Because God's ways are higher than man's ways, we must side with God. God has clearly stated that one man must marry one woman. It becomes problematic when we decide that man's laws are better than God's laws. The only way we can come to that conclusion is if we do not believe in God at all. After all, perfection is bound up in the idea of God.

Of course, some religious proponents of same-sex marriage might state that our *understanding* of God's laws is incorrect. God demonstrated the fact that He opposes same-sex marriage when He created Adam. God stated, "It is not good that the man should be alone."[3] He then created a person who would be suitable for Adam. This partnering that God began with remains His model for mankind. Genesis 5:2 begins with these words, "Male and female created He them; and *blessed them*" (italics mine). When it comes to marriage, God only blesses the one-man-one-woman arrangement that He instituted.

A relevant question here is as follows: Which gender did God create for Adam? Of course, God created a female, Eve, to be with Adam. God did not create a Steve, nor did God create Madam and Eve. God created a male and female to start the human race; that was part of His plan. We must not tamper with that arrangement.

Male and female created He them; and blessed them. —Genesis 5:2

Jesus Christ, the Son of God, repeated God the Father concerning the very beginning of the creation of humanity. In Matthew 19:4–5, Jesus stated, "Have you not read, that He which made them at the beginning made them male and female … for this cause shall a man leave father and mother, and shall cleave to his wife: and the two shall be one flesh." Thus, the first book of the New Testament affirms the fact that one man must only be with one woman.

Be Fruitful and Multiply

A second implicit directive of God regarding homosexuality comes in the form of His commandment to "be fruitful and multiply."[4] The only way to complete this directive in a natural way is to pair a man with a woman. The man provides the seed for life, and the woman provides the womb (the incubator). Two men can provide the seeds but not the incubator; two women can provide two incubators but no seeds. A gay man has no place to house a seed; consequently, the seed withers. A gay woman lacks a seed to bring forth life.

Both sexes must be together to procreate. Of course, we can do it man's way, but is that way God's way? Because it takes a father and a mother to make a child, it stands to reason that this arrangement is best throughout the life of the child. Society is taking what God created and attempting to usurp God's design and rules.

What would become of humanity if no one joined with the opposite sex? In the final book of the Old Testament, Malachi 2:15 mentions that one reason God granted a man for his wife is so they can produce godly offspring. The Lord mandates that such a union must take place within the confines of marriage. In the first book of the Old Testament (Genesis 2:24), God states that a man should leave his mother and father to be with his wife. It is worth noting that a man should have a mother and a father, not two mothers or two fathers. The main point is that a man should be united to a woman, not another man.

In the New Testament, Paul reiterates the verse from Genesis, noting that the two shall be one flesh (1 Corinthians 6:16). Two men or two women can never become one flesh in God's definition. Paul even refers to the union as a symbol of Christ and the church. He states, "For the husband is the head of the wife, even as Christ is the head of the church."[5] The same-sex marriage smacks of blasphemy when considering the fact that Christ is the head of the church.

An issue that naturally arises in any relationship is one of authority. The Bible names the husband as the spiritual head, just as Christ is the head of the church. In a same-sex marriage, who would have the spiritual authority? There can only be confusion unless one of the partners has taken the role of the leader voluntarily, but then the partnership is just mimicking the model that God has instituted. We cannot take just a piece of what God says and leave the rest undone. We must follow God's blueprint for marriage, especially in regards to something as important as creation.

God also commanded that we populate the earth after the great flood. "And you, be ye fruitful, and multiply; bring forth abundantly in the earth, and multiply therein."[6] Both when God started the human race and when He restarted it, the Lord issued the decree to procreate. The only way to procreate is to join one man and one woman.

Modern technology has brought about artificial insemination, whereby we can join a man's sperm with a woman's egg and create life in the laboratory. Using this practice in the attempt to create children for a same-sex marriage is truly infringing on God's "copyright" and using it to establish a family that God never intended.[7] Mankind has often attempted to use God for its own purposes. Likewise, mankind has often disrespected God when it disagreed with Him. To illustrate this point, contemplate the difference between outlawing prayer in schools and praying to God for rain.

What are society's laws against copyright infringement? Lawsuits ensue when someone violates another's intellectual property. God does not operate in our courtroom environments; however, He does hold His own court. If we do not want to be on the wrong side of God's justice, we must steer away from legalizing what God has condemned.

Besides procreation, there are other reasons God decreed one man must be with one woman. God stated the two sexes would be one flesh, and man with man or woman with woman cannot complete this spiritual feat. 1 Corinthians 6:12–20 speaks about the spiritual component of marriage. Verse 17 states, "But he that is joined unto the Lord is one spirit." The next phrase after that commands us to flee sexual immorality. Homosexuality is one example of sexual immorality, which means that same-sex sexual relations can never lead to spiritual union with the Lord in heaven. Verse 18 goes on to mention that whoever commits sexual immorality is sinning against his or her own body. Consider all the sexual diseases caused by sexual immorality that we are bombarded with.

There are other reasons God designed us the way that He did. This is where faith comes in. Remember: "Faith is trust without reservation."[8] We live by what we know, even when we do not know all the reasons. We trust and rely wholly on God and His Word, which tells us not to practice homosexuality.

Judgment of Great Transgression

Paul also addresses the subject of homosexuality in Colossians 3:5. He tells us to kill off our own evil desires, including sexual immorality. In the next verse, he prophesies that judgment and wrath are coming due to these things. In Romans 1:18, Scripture tells us that "the wrath of God is revealed from heaven against all ungodliness and unrighteousness of men."

Not only is the wrath of God coming because of the sin of homosexuality, but also because of all sinfulness. Homosexuality among those who claim to be part of the Body of Christ is especially repugnant because (as stated at the end of the eighteenth verse) "they hold the truth in unrighteousness." Many proponents of gay marriage proclaim the truth of God while living openly in abominable relationships.

God's church, which is entrusted with *the* truth, should not be living in unrighteousness. This type of open and defiant sin is described as "the great transgression" in Psalm 19:13. This is the final and most offensive sin mentioned in verses 12 and 13, wherein Scripture spells out the four types of sin in descending order. The least offensive sins deal with mistakes or errors. This category of sin is a big reason why the prayer the Lord taught us how to pray—"The Lord's Prayer"—should be prayed daily. In it, we find the following phrase: "Forgive us our sins." The apostle, John, also refers to these errors in his first epistle (in 1:8): "If we say that we have no sin, we deceive ourselves, and the truth is not in us." At times, we do not realize until after the fact that we have sinned. At times, we don't even realize we have sinned.

The second type of sin deals with secret or hidden faults. We are guilty of this when we sin (and know that we have sinned), but we try to keep the sins hidden from others. Our hearts and minds tell us that we have done wrong, but the conscience of our spirits is ashamed or afraid others will find out. Requesting forgiveness for this type of sin is a must if we are to maintain a pure conscience before God and man. Also, once we cross the boundary between this category of sin and the next, we are seriously endangering our relationships with God.

A boundary is crossed when we begin to sin without attempting to hide the sins from anyone. Worse yet, we cross that boundary when we are no longer ashamed of our sins. The Bible calls this presumptuous or willful sin. The psalmist begs God to help himself overcome this third category of sin so that he can remain upright. After all, the continued practice of this third category of sin may lead to the final area of sin.

We must steer away from this current trend of legalizing what God has condemned.

The final, and worst, type of sin in Psalm 19:13 is termed "the great transgression." I do not believe that the great transgression is limited to one sin. I do believe that the sin of homosexuality is one of them, though, considering the fact that the Lord calls it an abomination. The stages of homosexuality, or any other sin, typically follow the worsening pattern I have described.

First, the sin is considered an error, and then a secret fault, and then a willful sin, and then a great transgression. When God calls something evil and others claim that that same thing is good or godly, I believe they have crossed over into great transgression.[9]

Incidentally, Psalm 19 and the beginning of the book of Romans teach that God has revealed Himself and His ways to all of mankind—first, through what He has created (Psalm 19:1–6; Romans 1); second, via our conscience (Psalm 19:7–11; Romans 2); and finally, through His Son, Jesus Christ (Psalm 19:14; Romans 3). Moreover, by all of these means—and especially through God's Word, the Bible, and Jesus Christ—we have been warned. And if we living in accordance with the truth, we will earn a great reward.[10]

Continuing in Romans 1:19–25, God reveals that He has clearly shown all of us what His ways are. According to the twentieth verse, God's one man with one woman truth is evident by how He made the first couple. Some have rejected God's ways and "changed the truth of God into a lie" (verse 25), and due to this fact, God gave them over to the vile affection of homosexual relations (verses 26–27). In the end, each of us will believe what we will, but only the truth will remain eternally. We will all know at the final judgment, and of course, we will be able to guess intelligently what that truth is as the last days unfold.

The remainder of the Bible chapter that contains one of the definitive verses on God's view of homosexuality, Leviticus 18:22, goes on to explain the effects of allowing these and similar practices to transpire. God relates to the people that He drove the previous inhabitants out of the land because of these detestable practices. He states that, in the event of similar behavior, the land will vomit them out, too. That punishment is a little less severe than that delivered in Sodom and Gomorrah. Jude 7 encapsulates the tragedy of Sodom and Gomorrah by noting the sin and the resulting judgment.

The United States of America may face a similar judgment. Many catastrophes and tragedies have befallen our country over the past several years, more so than in many of the preceding decades. New diseases and viruses have arisen that surpass those of preceding generations. Do you believe the weather catastrophes of the past several years have been coincidental? Terrorism, also, is a scourge that will seemingly never fade away. Will America ever escape the drumbeats of war?

Sodom and Gomorrah

Sodom and Gomorrah were the infamous cities in Genesis that God destroyed because their sin was very grievous. The nineteenth chapter of Genesis describes a disgusting incident that occurred when the angels from the Lord went there to warn Lot and his family of the cities' impending doom. Ezekiel 16:49–50 adds much to that true tale by enumerating the sins of Sodom and why those sins were the cause of the city's ruin.

The first sin mentioned was the same sin that Lucifer was guilty of before he fell from heaven: namely, pride. Ezekiel next mentions that Sodom had an abundance of bread and idleness but did not take care of the poor and needy. The final sin, mentioned in the fiftieth verse, fell into the final, damning category of sin: the cities had committed an abomination before God. This abomination was likely the sin of homosexuality because it was not mentioned before in Ezekiel 16, and we know how God feels about this sin.[11]

The prophet, Isaiah, speaks of Sodom and Gomorrah at the beginning of his prophecies from the Lord. He specifically refers to the religious practices and evil deeds carried about by the people in these cities.[12] It appears that the inhabitants of Sodom and Gomorrah wanted to practice their sins while maintaining a form of godliness.

There exist people in America who want to maintain their gay lifestyles while maintaining their roles in God's flock. These people belong to something they call the gay church. Isaiah 3:9 and beyond reveals the fate of those who practice the sin of Sodom without repenting. God's view of this is best expressed by Isaiah 1:18, "Come now, and let us reason together … though your sins be as scarlet, they shall be as white as snow." Remember that the sin of Sodom and Gomorrah was not just the abomination of homosexuality, but also their unwillingness to "learn to do well; seek judgment, relieve the oppressed, defend the fatherless, plead for the widow."[13] Starting with Isaiah

3:10, we learn that all will go well with the righteous, but not so well with the wicked.

There is a group of gay churches that claim that such churches are just as much a part of the Body of Christ as any other; they claim that same-sex marriage is okay. These groups purport to hold and proclaim the Word of God while living in abominable sin. True belief in God results in a changed lifestyle. Some of Jesus' first words when He entered public ministry were as follows: "Repent ye, and believe the Gospel."[14] Repentance comes before or at belief, and repentance signifies a changed heart and mind and way of living.[15]

There are many other believers (and even ministers) who live a life of sin while actively involved in God's household of faith; however, the gay churches go well beyond those sins and attempt to highlight their sinfulness. The gayness of the world is the sadness of God. I do not want to imagine how God views the gaying of the church. It could be that, in His eyes, these two things are mutually exclusive.

4

Sodom and Gomorrah: A Revised History

If God wrote a book, would you read it? We have great authors in the world today, and there have been countless great authors throughout history. Some people love to read and will read anything about anything. Some like to read and focus primarily on certain passions. Some people read very little, if at all. If God wrote something, whether we have read a thousand books or none, that writing should be read by all. If God were to write a book right now, what a book that book would be!

I can imagine a book that stated on its cover that the author was God. That book would be an incredible book. It might tell us who we are, where we came from, what we are doing on earth, why we are here. It would surely be on the best-seller list in every country. Of course, it would be translated into every known language. In fact, I'm sure it would be the best seller of all time. If God wrote a book, one could only begin to imagine the fantastic things that would be inside of it. What great wonders, words, stories, histories, and viewpoints would be given to us! God might tell us some things that are so beautiful that we could hardly contain ourselves. God might tell us things that, even if we experienced them with our own senses, we would still declare them to be unbelievable.

The stories God could tell would be captivating, shocking, and more appealing than those any human could tell. Everyone would be extremely interested in God's opinions on all topics. If God were to write a book, the writings would speak to and encompass all of humanity, every possible aspect of it. God's writing would speak to all humans from the beginning of time to beyond all tomorrows.

God, it seems to me, would be concerned with every part of what was happening on this planet. God would answer questions on every imaginable topic in His book. God would write in such a way that anyone could understand Him; although, because the writing came from a higher life form, we might wrestle with some of the ideas. Humanity would be able to comprehend what God wrote, yet there would be enough in God's words to keep us busy for a lifetime. Such would be the writing of

God: beautiful to read, understood by children, debated by scholars, and loved by all.

Of course, God did write a book. It is called the Bible. Humans wrote the words down, but do not be mistaken about it: the words from the Bible actually came from the mind of God.[1] A secretary may write the words down, but the words come from the author. The book of Genesis is the first book in the Bible, and it tells of the very beginning of the human race. In the nineteenth chapter of Genesis, we are told the historical account of two cities that tested God on the same subject that America is testing God on today.

Genesis 19 tells the sad story of Sodom and Gomorrah. What if history had not gone entirely as Genesis 19 described it? What if the cities of Sodom and Gomorrah had not been totally destroyed and wiped off the face of the earth? History might have been different. Beginning from the climax in the twenty-fourth verse—"Then the LORD rained upon Sodom and upon Gomorrah brimstone and fire from the LORD out of heaven"—things would be different.

A revised and fictional history might read like this: fortunately for the Sodomites and inhabitants of Gomorrah, they had prepared themselves well for the fiery rain. They took a page out of the Holy Bible, from the story of the Tower of Babel, wherein God states that, because the people were all as one, nothing they put their minds to would be withheld from them.[2] Just prior to the rain from God, they completed and deployed an atmospheric shield. Although the brimstone and fire fractured parts of the shield and destroyed small sections of the cities, the shield held up remarkably well.

From then on, Sodom and Gomorrah began to propagate their form of sexuality. They began to legislate their agenda, following the lead of the abortion industry. Even though mankind enjoyed their lives, they wanted to rid themselves of any semblance of God in "their" world. The followers of the Sodom and Gomorrah philosophy wanted to show their Creator that they could get along just fine without Him, similar to the builders of the Tower of Babel. Though God informed them of their genesis with Adam and Eve, they preferred two Adams and two Eves together in same-sex marriages. Unfortunately, their plan did not go well. Within one hundred years of forcibly mandating only gay marriage, the population grew old and died off, leaving the earth devoid of humans.

Gay marriage, in effect, makes God sad. After all, His most prized creation, mankind, cannot procreate in a world of only gay marriage. As the Tower of Babel was the rebellion of mankind against the direction of God to fill the earth, likewise, the homosexual lifestyle makes the mandate of God to be fruitful and multiply impossible. These wicked philosophies come from the father of lies, Satan. In a variation of a play in his despicable playbook, Satan claimed that God did not really state that marriage should only be between one man and one woman. Two legendary authors have written fantastic fiction about other lies instigated by Satan. J. R. R. Tolkien, in *The Silmarillion*, the prequel to *The Lord of the Rings* and *The Hobbit,* tells of Morgoth (or Melkor); and C. S. Lewis, in *The Chronicles of Narnia,* writes about the White Witch (or Jadis).

Of course, the revised history I outlined would be a preposterous turn of events; I only told it to highlight my point. It is possible that Sodom and Gomorrah created laws legalizing homosexual marriage and granted to those couples the same privileges that are bestowed upon traditional marriages. This is the same fixation that America is falling under today.

We should not treat gays unfairly or discriminate against them on a personal level. Similarly, no one should treat them with disrespect or without dignity. But at the same time, we should not make the law of the land what God has stated is wrong. David Wilkerson, in his prophetic work, *America's Last Call,* writes about Sodom and Gomorrah. He also writes about another disturbing homosexual encounter in Judges (the nineteenth and twentieth chapters): "The flash point for the judgment of God comes at the very hour a militant homosexual spirit rises up and attacks what is divine and holy."[3]

We should not make the law of the land what God has stated is wrong.

Homosexuality is a sin like the others, but one notable aspect of it is that the public and legal acceptance of it will usher in the end, in one form or another. In what appears to be a story about America, Romans 9:29, quoting from Isaiah 1:9, states that, unless God had left the nation a small remnant, the nation would have been like Sodom and Gomorrah. Isaiah 1:21 speaks of how the "faithful city became a harlot." It was previously full of justice and righteousness, but it became filled with murder (including abortion).

Psalm 107:33–34 indicates that God will dry up the land and turn "fruitful land into barrenness" … all due to the "wickedness of them that dwell therein." Abortion is definitely an abhorrent attack on God's most precious creation, mankind. Abortion was instigated by the one who fell from grace in heaven and came to earth to kill and destroy us. If allowed to play out, God's most precious creation could be terminated by gay marriage, abortion, and other practices decried by God. If that happens, we must blame Satan's lies.

5

The Prenatal Holocaust

I will not write much on this topic because it is not exactly the topic of this book. Plus, many others have written extensively and eloquently about it already. Still, I want to say a little because the subject somewhat relates to the gaying of America. In addition to the killing of the millions of created, yet unborn, babies, I believe that God even grieves all the little ones who will never be born because society condones same-sex marriage.

We should place God and His ways above what we want, need, or even deserve. Compared to same-sex marriage and pro-choice stances, all other issues pale. I am sure that God is less concerned about how well off and comfortable we are than with how many of His precious ones are being cut up and discarded daily.

If only we would look to God for his benefits and blessings instead of continuing in our evil ways. When will we allow all the little ones to participate in God's benefits and blessings? We should focus less on temporal matters and more on eternal matters. The world passes away, but one who does the will of God abides forever.[1] God told us that heaven and earth would pass away, but the Word of God will last forever.[2]

As human beings, we will last forever, including the next life. Thus, after the Lord, our focus should be on humanity and the weakest, smallest, and most vulnerable. We ought to look beyond the clouds of temporary matters and see the heavens of eternal matters that exist beyond. Past the clouds is the Son of Righteousness! If only more could see Him.

God even grieves all the little ones who will never be born because society condones same-sex marriage.

Abortion is a crime against God and our fellow human beings, and it is especially hideous in this technologically advanced age because we can see the little ones on sonogram screens. I want to be on the side of God and

His Holy Word and end this tragedy. The American presidential election of 2012 was, in my estimation, a referendum on God: the lines and sides were clearly delineated. The proponents on each side of these major issues made their points very clear.

The people who chose the man who refuses to fight for the lives of the unborn and, months before, endorsed gay marriage, have undermined God's mandates. The president basically stated, "Did God really say men could not marry men, women could not marry women?" He essentially asked, "Did God really say life began at conception?" We can't go further back than our genesis without facing our Creator. Once we reach that point, humanity might believe that it can forge its own rules regardless of what God says.

Mother Teresa had this to say on the subject of abortion: "Human rights are not a privilege conferred by government. They are every human being's entitlement by virtue of his humanity. The right to life does not depend, and must not be declared to be contingent, on the pleasure of anyone else, not even a parent or a sovereign."[3] A Christian artist, Phil Keaggy, sang these lyrics:

Who will speak up for the little ones?
Helpless and half-abandoned.

They've got the right to choose life
They don't want to lose.[4]

Many do not recognize the God of the Bible as the Creator, and many do not recognize Jesus Christ. Jesus was the one who said, "My Kingdom is not of this world." Today, I rejoice that believers "are not of this world." I continue to be saddened by the stand America is taking. No matter how mighty the country is, if it is faulty at its foundation, it will crumble. The killing of unborn, innocent children and the legalization of same-sex marriage is an affront to the One who made us.

Children remain one of the greatest gifts a person can receive during his or her lifetime. God gives us little ones that we have the opportunity to shape. We must not be lax in accomplishing that which we have been tasked with doing. All too often, we hear of children who endure the shortcomings of a parent or guardian, and those facts usually come to light only after many months or years of suffering.

Our children reflect what we put into them; let's put the good things of this life into them instead of the bad. If you are blessed with the ability to procreate, I only hope you are also blessed with the ability to raise and train a child in the right way.[5] Children have been given to us as a heritage.[6]

If we expect our children to honor us, we must honor their rights. First of all, we must honor their right to life. After that, we must provide a decent and fulfilling life for them. Children will, in large measure, produce what we have produced in them. Kids reflect those who raise them. What goes in, comes out: it is an observation that is often accurate in regard to child rearing.

If a parent wishes to see his or her outward appearance, he or she need only look into a mirror; however, if a parent wants to see his or her inward appearance, he or she should look at the behavior of his or her child. In most cases, a person's children manifest telltale expressions of that person's character. Consider the untold instances in your own life when you've heard someone say, "He acts just like his father," for example.

The way in which we bring up our children forms a mark that we leave on society. When the children see us doing something, they are prone to behave in the same manner. If we act kind to them, they learn to behave kindly. If we show patience toward them, they exhibit patience toward others. The exhibition of these standards cannot be an infrequent occurrence; they must be demonstrated on a regular basis. The proper treatment of children should begin before birth, from the very moment of conception.

Formerly, when speaking or writing on this topic, I would state that anyone could produce a child, but it takes real men and women to raise children the right way. Although I still believe that statement, I must qualify it by saying that, in this day and age, not just anyone can create a child. It takes one man and one woman to produce a child. Beginning with that foundation, we must defend God's edicts. There is still time for repentance, but the fuse is approaching its end. Keep in mind that Jesus can forgive us and justify us just as if we had never sinned.

6

The Decay and Fall of the American Empire

In May of 2012, President Barack Obama became the first American president to publicly favor same-sex marriage. His support of gay marriage ushered in a new era in this country and in the spiritual world. Seemingly, we hear about some new development in the advancement of the homosexual agenda on a weekly basis. With the Supreme Court of the United States hearing arguments on same-sex marriage in 2013, it is likely inevitable that they will one day approve it or turn a blind eye to it and allow it to proceed. The voters of California voted not to recognize same-sex marriage, but a state court deemed the resulting law unconstitutional. By not allowing an appeal to the lower court ruling in California's Proposition 8, the Supreme Court of the United States effectively let that lower court's ruling stand, allowing same-sex marriage in California. Sadly, one activist court overruled the will of the people.

June 26, 2013: Hell Will Celebrate This Day

On the same day, the Supreme Court struck down the federal *Defense of Marriage Act* (*DOMA*), which had defined marriage as a bond between one man and one woman. The judicial system continues to join governments across the country in legislating, legalizing, and mandating immorality. Many states are being forced to go against God's explicit laws and legally recognize homosexual marriage.

Signed into law in 1996, DOMA prohibited the federal recognition of any marriage other than one between a man and a woman. Because DOMA was deemed unconstitutional, the federal government is forced to recognize any gay marriage in states where it is legal, bestowing the same rights and benefits granted to God-sanctioned marriage.

Though I am not a conspiracy theorist, I am nonetheless struck by the case that led to the destruction of DOMA. *Windsor v. United States* should not have been elevated to the Supreme Court of the United States, much less decided the way it was. Edith Windsor, the plaintiff, won the tax-based case, and the United States, the defendant, agreed with her win. Thus, the Supreme Court should not have received the case. The sinister method in which it was contrived seems eerily demonic. In dissent, Justice Antonin Scalia commented, "We have no power to decide this case, and even if we did, we have no power under the Constitution to invalidate this democratically adopted legislation [*DOMA*]." Later in his opinion, with Chief Justice John Roberts and Justice Clarence Thomas joining, Justice Scalia stated,

> What the petitioner United States asks us to do in the case before us is exactly what the respondent Windsor asks us to do; not to provide relief from the judgment below but to say that that judgment was correct. And the same was true in the Court of Appeals: Neither party sought to undo the judgment for Windsor, and so that court should have dismissed the appeal (just as we should dismiss) for lack of jurisdiction. Since both parties agreed with the judgment of the District Court for the Southern District of New York, the suit should have ended there. The further proceedings have been a contrivance, having no object in mind except to elevate a District Court judgment that has no precedential effect in other courts, to one that has precedential effect throughout the Second Circuit, and then

(in this Court) precedential effect throughout the United States.

We have never before agreed to speak—to "say what the law is"—where there is no controversy before us. In the more than two centuries that this Court has existed as an institution, we have never suggested that we have the power to decide a question when every party agrees with both its nominal opponent and the court below on that question's answer. The United States reluctantly conceded that at oral argument.1

Referring to the moral impact of the ruling, the Chaplain Alliance for Religious Liberty, an organization representing more than 2,000 chaplains who actively serve the armed forces, expressed disappointment. The group was upset that the Supreme Court chose to strike down the definition of marriage for the purposes of federal law found in the *Defense of Marriage Act*. A brief excerpt from their statement reads as follows: "Most of the faith groups in our country firmly hold that marriage is the union of one man and one woman. They strongly believe that children deserve to know their mother and father."[2]

Less to Celebrate

Early in 2013, a US Senator, Rob Portman, supported gay marriage only when his son came out. Portman, a former opponent of same-sex marriage, wavered when his son revealed to him that he was gay. Should we ever forsake God's ways, even for the sake of our own family? In my estimation, we ought to support God's ways over our loved ones' ways. If a family member says he or she is gay, we should still love that person unconditionally and treat him or her with respect and dignity. But we should be faithful to God's Word and continue to instruct our loved one to be righteous. We should always accept people, even if we don't approve of everything they do.

In May of 2013, a professional basketball player, Jason Collins, became the first athlete to publicly announce his gayness. He was treated by many as a hero. This praise for what God calls an abomination is precisely what God was referring to in Isaiah 5:20 and Malachi 2:17 when he noted that humans were capable of calling evil good. In September 2011, the U.S. military changed the already inclusive "don't ask don't tell" homosexual policy to one of open acceptance. This societal acceptance of gay marriage may be one of the final straws of the undoing of America.

As of this writing, sixteen American states allow gay marriage: California, Connecticut, Delaware, Hawaii, Iowa, Maine, Maryland, Massachusetts, Minnesota, New Hampshire, New Jersey, New Mexico, New York, Rhode Island, Washington, and Vermont. The District of Columbia also allows gay marriage. In Genesis, the story of Abraham and the cities of Sodom and Gomorrah is told. Abraham begged for these two ungodly cities to be spared. Destruction was decreed in part (if not primarily) because of the cities' acceptance of homosexuality.

Abraham began his prayer, or intercession, for Sodom and Gomorrah by asking God, "What if there be fifty righteous within the city: will You also destroy and not spare the place for the fifty righteous that are therein?"[3] God told him that He would not destroy the cities if there were fifty righteous within the city. Abraham then lowered the righteous total to forty-five, and then he lowered the total to forty. He went on until he questioned whether God would refrain from destroying the cities for the sake of just ten righteous people. God said that He would not.

To me, it is no small coincidence that the United States of America has the same number of states as the number of righteous people that Abraham first petitioned God about. Will God deal with or execute judgment on

America if forty states do not allow gay marriage? What about thirty-five? Twenty-five? Ten? Will God deal with this country once the total of states that forbid same-sex marriage dips below ten? It may be that this is the path that we are on.

Will God deal with this country once the total of states that forbid same-sex marriage dips below ten?

It is possible that God is looking down on America to see whether fewer than ten states will behave righteously by banning gay marriage. Abraham was counting righteous people, I am counting American states. If this comparison holds true, when forty-one or more states legalize same-sex marriage, God will finally and fully judge the many sins of the United States of America.

After the great flood in Genesis, God established a covenant with mankind that He would never again cause a great flood that would destroy all flesh. It is ironic that the sign that God gave for this covenant is the same symbol that the gay community has chosen for itself: the rainbow. If the prophetic prediction of this book holds true, the rainbow will turn out to be mankind's symbol to God that humanity has utterly disregarded God's commandments. In essence, we will have mocked God's previous judgment of Sodom and Gomorrah with the sacrilegious use of the rainbow.

God says He did away with Sodom and Gomorrah because of their haughtiness and the abomination committed. These sins were occurring long before the cities were destroyed by fire.[4] Ezekiel 16:49–50 spells out a list of sins that Sodom was guilty of, which prompted the judgment of God. If we look across America today, we can easily observe the same list of sins mentioned in Genesis and Ezekiel. And the final one, the abomination, is being increasingly accepted in society and its laws.

If one accepts that the Bible is true, then one must accept that everything that is written in it is true. We cannot choose to believe parts of it that we think are suitable. To me, that would be like claiming that Jesus is only partly God. Jesus declared Himself to be God, so if He is not, Jesus must have been lying. I am sure there are not many people who believe Jesus was a liar. C. S. Lewis and Josh McDowell have a wonderful discussion about whether Jesus was Lord, liar, or lunatic.[5]

If we believe that the Bible, in its entirety, is true, we must accept that Sodom and Gomorrah were real places that were really destroyed by God. The sins that brought on God's judgment were really being committed there. The United States of America is following that same path. Of the sins that are spoken of in Sodom and Gomorrah, none could realistically be legislated except the final sin mentioned.

This societal acceptance of gay marriage may be the undoing of America.

It is not realistic in a democracy to outlaw pride, idleness, greed, or selfishness. I do not believe those sins were legislated against in Sodom and Gomorrah; however, it is possible that the sin of homosexuality was indeed legislated. It is a certainty that many Americans embrace the other sins for which Sodom and Gomorrah were judged. It is also a certainty that many live in the sin of homosexuality; however, when society dictates that this sin is legal, we will be on a slippery slope that culminates in God's judgment. Such legislation is tantamount to legislating pride, idleness, greed, selfishness, and any other behavior that God declares is sinful.

Jude 7 and 8 inform us that Sodom and Gomorrah gave themselves over to sexually immoral behavior and perversion. They were "set forth for an example, suffering the vengeance of eternal fire." The Pandora's box of homosexuality has been opened, and likely, there is no turning back. There is only a dread of coming judgment, as Jonathan Edwards preached in *Sinners in the Hands of an Angry God*.

This escalation of public acceptance of sinning is quickly becoming the story of our country. The homosexual issue, in particular, will allow mainstream society to be extremely critical of Christians, especially when some overly zealous and errant believers treat the homosexual community inappropriately. The errant Christians will be taken as our spokespeople, and the world will attack all believers because of their allegedly hateful and mean-spirited actions.

We all know about the governmental encroachment into our public and private lives. Common citizens are being monitored regularly in various ways. The case of a football player, Aaron Hernandez, highlights the use of satellites to track our every move. Recently, it came to light that the US Postal Service captures the image of every letter mailed out by every person within this country.

The National Security Agency's (NSA) intrusive public surveillance program has come into full view since late spring of 2013. Personal cell phone records have been adjudged to be accessible by law enforcement due to their public nature. According to officials, individuals choose to use public air space, which makes tapping into cell phones fair game.

One of the largest cities in our country, San Antonio, Texas, approved a measure in September of 2013 that bans anyone from serving in any official governmental capacity who has openly uttered a word against homosexuality. Several other threatening features have been adopted with this city ordinance. It was slightly modified during deliberations because concerned Christian citizens voiced their opposition, but it still passed largely intact.[6]

Mounted on many traffic intersections, and beginning to be installed on police vehicles, are video cameras that constantly photograph license plates to track the movement of vehicles. While preparing this manuscript, my own son was pulled over. Though he was going under the speed limit, following the flow of traffic, and seemingly obeying the law, the police officer nevertheless ran his license plate while they were driving and discovered that my son's insurance had expired three days earlier. The officer pulled him over and had the car towed away.

All of these steps make it easy for the government to monitor many phases of our lives. And these measures will eventually be used to incriminate Christians wrongfully. Believers in God who follow and declare God's unchanging laws to the world will one day be targets of their own government and fellow citizens. I believe that the trend toward public acceptance of homosexual marriage and similar laws will usher in this attack on Christians. All that is lacking is a leader who will not tolerate the laws of God and persecute Christians. Same-sex marriage will be the issue that causes Americans to accept and participate in the strong criticism of devout followers of God. American believers will be placed in the same situation as many believers in the rest of the world (see www.persecution.com for more information).

As George O. Wood, general superintendent of the Assemblies of God, wrote in his statement of the aforementioned *DOMA* ruling,

> It is especially disturbing that Justice Kennedy, in his majority opinion, identified "animus" against homosexuals as one motivating factor in the adoption of the Congressional Defense of Marriage Act. To apply the word "animus"

to those who hold to the view that marriage is reserved for a man and woman is an inflammatory accusation that ignores our principled arguments and demeans our motives.

You see this animus in Christians being labeled as haters, homophobes and bigots when the reverse is true. Humanitarian care and love for neighbor is a timeless value demonstrated daily by Christians. If the culture can dehumanize followers of Christ by attaching hateful labels to them, then it's only a matter of time until Christians are first marginalized for their faith, deprived of their 1st amendment rights, and ultimately persecuted.[7]

Already, in the United States, cases are beginning that underscore the new marginalizing of people who stand their pro-God ground. A judge in the state of New Mexico agreed with a plaintiff that sued a photographer for refusing to photograph a same-sex marriage. The photographer's defense was that her conscience, guided by Christian beliefs, would not allow such activity. In August of 2013, *Elane Photography v. Willock* was appealed to and upheld in the New Mexico Supreme Court.[8]

Effects of Same-Sex Marriage in Canada[9]

Consider Canada, which legalized gay marriage in 2003. Several lawsuits have occurred there that have detrimentally affected Christians. Manitoba marriage commissioners were notified in 2004 that they would be required to perform ceremonies for same-sex marriages or lose their licenses. Due to his Christian beliefs, a marriage commissioner in Saskatchewan refused to marry two men. He was fined by the Human Rights Tribunal.

In another case, a British Columbia educator had his teacher's license suspended for writing to a newspaper and describing the Christian perspective on homosexuality. That same teacher appeared before parliament as a witness during federal debate on same-sex marriage, and he received three more months of suspension. In the same region, in 2006, the Ministry of Education announced it would include mandatory "positive" lessons about homosexuality in every grade. Parents could not opt out of the classroom lessons, even though they were sensitive in nature. That same parental policy was in effect for all lessons involving homosexuality.

A church bishop in Calgary was threatened by the Customs and Revenue Agency in 2004 with the possible loss of his church's charitable tax exemption status because he wrote a letter to his congregation pointing out the possible error of a Catholic political leader. The bishop was telling his church that supporting same-sex marriage and abortion was wrong.

In 2005, in Saskatchewan, a tribunal charged a local man with hate speech because he was alleged to have "hurt the feelings" of several homosexuals. What did he do? He distributed a flyer warning people about the dangers of the gay lifestyle. A lifetime public speaking ban (if the subject was homosexuality) was imposed upon the man. The appeals court upheld the verdict, thus impeding his right to free speech. Early in 2013, the case was heard at the Canadian Supreme Court. The Campaign Life Coalition stated the following:

> A chilling decision is handed down by the court which many pro-family and free speech advocates regard as "a monumental blow against freedom of speech, opinion, and religion across the country." In effect, the court states that criticism of the homosexual lifestyle, can indeed be considered a "hate crime." The court rejects as a possible defence against a hate speech accusation, the traditional teaching of the Catholic Church to

"love the sinner but not the sin," ruling that when it comes to homosexual sex, criticism of "behavior" is to be deemed the same as an attack on homosexual persons. The judges even opine that truth is no defense. In effect, this court ruling outlaws public expression of biblical teaching against homosexual acts.[9]

In 2013, a Canadian Re/Max real estate agency fired an employee for publishing a flyer containing articles that promoted traditional family parental roles. Based on scientific findings, some articles claimed traditional heterosexual parenting over homosexual parenting was better for the children. Cases such as this highlight the discrimination levied against the rights of Christians to earn a living. (See the URL listed in the ninth note of this chapter for more examples of attacks on Christians.)

Called Out

Individual acceptance of—and even practice of—homosexuality is completely different from public policy acceptance of homosexuality. It is one thing to do what you as an individual want to do, but it is an entirely different matter to make it a law that everyone must recognize and accept gay rights and same-sex marriage as public policy. The nation of Judah carried out evil by allowing sodomites in the land; Kings Jehoshaphat and Asa "did that which was right in the eyes of the Lord" by removing the sodomites from the land.[10]

I fear for our country because many Americans seem to be in favor of, or at least ready to institutionalize, these wicked practices. I believe the American presidential election of 2012 was a referendum on God because Barack Obama, in a calculated decision, announced his position on gay marriage well before the election. I find it hard to believe that a majority of Americans did not know God's stance on same-sex relations. I am especially perplexed by President Obama's lack of insight into God's stance, considering the fact that he has proclaimed to be a Christian for many years. How could the leader of our country, knowing God's position on homosexuality, intentionally endorse what God calls wickedness and an abomination? Was he duped by the gay community into believing that God doesn't intend what He stated in Holy Scripture? During my research, I came across several sites devoted to promoting homosexuality. I also found several that attempted to legitimize its practice, even within the church.

We have not been called out of sin in order to fall back into it.

Some compelling arguments notwithstanding, the bottom line is that the historicity of traditional Christianity founded in Scripture, aided by fallacies in homosexual proponent thinking, wins out on this subject. I expect God to judge the sin of homosexuality as He does with all other sin. Pope Francis's remark about homosexuals seems to be swaying Catholics. He said, "If a person is gay and seeks the Lord and has good will, who am I to judge that person?" Jesus stated that He had not come to judge the world, but to save it. But He clarified that sentiment by stating that "the Word that I have spoken … shall judge."[11] Of course, only Jesus is able to save the world, which leaves our role as true Christians to pointing everyone to Jesus and His Word for salvation.

The term *gay church* is as much an oxymoron as the term *the church of practicing sinners*. In fact, the word *church* comes from the Greek word *ekklesia*, which means *the called out ones*. (The Spanish word for church is *iglesia*, which sounds very similar to the Greek word.) The church has been called out from the world and sinful living and into righteous living. We have not been called out of sin in order to fall back into it or to continue to practice sinful living. One of the key verses advising the church to continue assembling and provoking one another toward love and good works goes on to say, "For if we sin willfully after that we have received the knowledge of the truth … there remains but a certain fearful looking for of judgment and fire."[12]

Homosexuals are not called to come out of the closet and shake their fist at God, but rather to come out and confess their sin and repent, just as everyone must do. Paul was transformed from a persecutor of people into a better person, and John gave up his anger for love. We are, likewise, called to allow our lives to be transformed. There are no exceptions.

Civil Rights?

As mentioned in the introduction, on the surface, gay rights seem to be a civil and human rights issue. Why shouldn't people have the *right* to do as they please as long as they aren't hurting anyone else? What does it really matter if two men or two women want to live together in matrimony? As an American, it may sound perfectly fine and legitimate; however, this is not an issue of civil or human rights. It is an issue of the "right"eousness of God.

Sin is sin, no matter how it is cloaked, no matter how it appears to us as humans.

The United States of America is succumbing to the question that Satan posed to Adam and Eve at the beginning of creation, "Did God really say…?"[13] Just as with our ancestors, Adam and Eve, it is a basic function of humanity to debate. In the book of Genesis, it was a question of eating—what a seemingly harmless proposition. Why shouldn't Adam and Eve be allowed to eat the fruit? Fruit is a natural and very healthy food. God even made fruit so that we could eat it and be healthy. What, then, was the problem? The fact is, God told Adam and Eve not to eat from that particular tree.

Today, why shouldn't humanity be allowed to fulfill its basic sexual necessities? After all, it was God who made us sexual creatures, and some of us yearn for the same sex. Even though we can live without sex, that is not the way God designed humanity. The Golden Rule even requires that we do unto others as we would have them do unto us. The second greatest command is to love your neighbor as you love yourself. In light of these two directives, why would we deprive our fellow citizens of choosing whomever they want to marry?

The reason we must stick with traditional marriage can be found in the first and very greatest command: Jesus stated that we must love God with all our heart, soul, mind, and strength.[14] How do we show our support of and love for God and His Holy Word in a practical manner? In a word, we obey Him. In the third chapter of this book, we discussed God's commandments in regards to homosexuality. Obedience to God also includes fulfilling the Ten Commandments.[15] The first four of the Ten Commandments focus on how we can go about showing our love for God. The final six of the Ten Commandments focus on how we can show love toward our fellow human beings. We fulfill the second greatest commandment to love our neighbor as ourselves by living by these final six commandments. Within these Ten Commandments, God has indicated His priorities.

The Priorities of God

Many who profess to be sincere Christians are so wrapped up in this world that they cannot determine God's priorities. God's priorities are based on eternal matters, and all eternal priorities proceed from God. The Bible tells us that God's Word is eternal, and that His human creation, once conceived, will likewise live forever. If eternal matters are God's priorities and the Bible is eternal, what proceeds from God's eternal Word, the Bible, is a priority.

If this nation continues to turn its back on God's priorities, we are destined for an unpleasant end. Gay marriage and abortion are definitely not the only issues in this country, but they ought to be the top of the list. Most voters choose a particular candidate based on what that candidate believes, promises to do, and holds as priorities. If Christians are not voting based on God's eternal Word and what is best for the life of God's most precious creation, humanity, we are in error.

Loving one's neighbor includes loving one's homosexual neighbor.

As God loves and respects all people, I love and respect all people, including gay people. I do not fear them. I am not a homophobe, nor am I prejudiced against them. I do not look down on them or hate them, even though they are sinning. After all, we are all sinners. We were all in that same sinner-not-yet-saved-by-grace boat once. As God condemns their behavior, so do I. But I do not condemn who they are as people. Jesus gave His life for every one of us, and God calls us to reciprocate His Love by laying down our life for others.[16]

The major problem arises when, as a nation, we legally mandate the acceptance of the gay lifestyle. America has, year after year, removed itself from God's favor by rejecting God's priorities and accepting evil as good. Americans appear to have turned the corner by living physically healthier lives, but on the moral and spiritual front, we are turning downward. What should Christians do regarding this downturn?

7

What Should We Then Do?

What should we do in response to the gaying of America? Hopefully, it is clear by now that what we should *not* do is condemn our fellow humans who are involved in this sin. Many gay people believe, or want to believe, that they were made gay and have no choice but to remain homosexual. Remember that at the fall of mankind in Eden, along with our spirit dying, our bodies, minds, emotions, and many other things were corrupted. None of us is perfect, so there is some area or issue in all of us that has problems. Everyone should reconcile their whole being with our Maker and His instructions.

If everyone knew what everyone else was up against, what a world we would have. There would be so much more understanding, concern, production, accountability, etc. That's how God does it! That's why He can be so patient with us, so understanding, considerate, and forgiving:

He knows all that we are up against. We ought to at least make an effort to understand what each of our neighbors is up against.

We must be more understanding of what gay people, and all other people, are dealing with. If we are not willing to learn to better understand their situation, we should at least avoid putting them down. They are part of humanity, as much as everyone else is. And because no one is without some sort of sin, no one should throw stones. One of the most recognized accounts of the compassion and wisdom of Jesus involves someone involved in sexual sin, just as we are discussing now. We should oft repeat the famous words of Jesus: "Neither do I condemn you; go, and sin no more."[1]

What are we to do with all the biblical passages that condemn the sin of homosexuality? They are clearly written for us in black and white. The best response I know came from a local pastor. The pastor counseled his wife during a time of trial and said, "When dealing with the black and white, don't forget about the red."[2] When we are confronted with obvious commandments, we must never forget about the shed blood of Jesus Christ. As the old refrain goes, "Oh the blood of Jesus, Oh the blood of Jesus, Oh the blood of Jesus, it washes white as snow."

Remember that the Bible is a spiritual book to be understood first in the spirit. For a person whose spirit is not born again, it is unlikely that they will be able to discern God's Word. Being born again is a prerequisite to begin to fully understand God's ways. Thus, we must pray that this rebirth experience takes place so that unbelievers can gain spiritual understanding and mental comprehension. This is the true responsibility of the Church; the Church should not condemn gay people. We must allow the Holy Spirit of God to bring conviction of sin, righteousness, and judgment into the spirit and soul of the unbeliever.[3]

God is so patient with us because He knows all that we are up against.

Remember that God instituted the Church so it would love all and preach the truth, not condemn people. "Love your neighbor as yourself" is the most quoted Old Testament verse in the New Testament; it is repeated eight times.[4] In fact, this Old Testament reference is found in the chapter that appears right after God's view of homosexuality is elucidated.[5] The church should reach out more to the whole LGBT community and shine the light of Jesus into that dark world.

When Jesus told us to love our neighbor, He was not excluding our homosexual neighbors. One of Jesus' neighbors was the adulterous woman caught in the act.[6] Jesus practiced what He preached. The woman was his neighbor, and He treated her the way we ought to treat all of our neighbors. We should not condone the sin, but we should love the person caught in the sin. I am sure we can find a way to react the way that Jesus did.

The Example of Abraham

Earlier we looked briefly at the example of Abraham and here is more detail. Looking back at Sodom and Gomorrah, we can see how the foremost believer of that day reacted to the news of the behavior in those cities. Genesis 18:16–33 relates the story of how the Lord notified Abraham of the coming judgment on Sodom and Gomorrah. Once the representatives of God left Abraham's house, Abraham "stood yet before the Lord." What was Abraham's response when he learned how God was planning to judge those wicked cities? Did he begin to heap condemnation upon them? No. Did he begin to berate them? No.

Abraham began to intercede, to pray, for the inhabitants of the cities. Yes, he immediately began to pray for them. He was bold enough to put himself on the line with the Lord for that wicked generation. Abraham begged the Lord no fewer than eight times to spare those people. He insightfully queried, "Shall not the Judge of all the earth do right?"[7] God declared that Abraham would command his children and his other descendants to keep the way of the Lord.[8] Abraham showed us what the way of the Lord was: he prayed and pled for Sodom and Gomorrah. We must also plead for our nation.

Intercession is truly taking care of God's business. As a child, Jesus stated that He must be about His Father's business (Luke 2:49). Unfortunately, it takes most of us years to realize that the purpose of life is to do the same. Even those who are believers in God spend many days occupied with errant tasks, or busy-ness. I remember when this idea first dawned on me many years ago: I tried to write out the word *business* so that it would be pronounced *busy-ness*. I realized that if I followed the normal English rules and replaced the *y* with an *i*, that the word would be spelled and pronounced *business*. We may see our busy-ness as God's business, but God may have a different opinion. True intercession before God is being about God's business in the same way that Abraham was.

When it comes to homosexuals, we should follow the renewed Apostle John's example and show less thunder and more love. The Word of God mandates that we hate sin, but God also commands us to love sinners. The sin of homosexuality warrants our thunder, but homosexuals warrant our love.

Homosexuality warrants our thunder, but homosexuals warrant our love.

If any person would have the right or obligation to condemn others, Abraham, the father of our faith, might be that one. Why did he not take the opportunity to flaunt his relationship with the God of the universe (according to Genesis 18:17–19)? Abraham already knew the lessons about love and consideration of others that Jesus verbalized centuries later.

Also, just before he prayed for Sodom and Gomorrah, Abraham doubted and even questioned God's wisdom on a certain matter (see Genesis 17:15-18). Abraham was well aware of his shortcomings and fallible humanity. How could he condemn others when he knew he was also a sinner? This really points once again to humility.

All things work together for good, even our mistakes. When God steps into our lives, there will be transformation. You cannot ask the God of creation, the world, the universe to come into your life and doubt you will be changed!

Problems in life come up, and we don't know how everything works together, but somehow it does (Romans 8:28 and Mark 4:26). God is in the business of transformation, so when He steps into a situation, things change. Some biblical examples of this are as follows:

Abraham doubted, and he is called the father of our faith.

Jacob deceived and took, and God called him Israel (*the prince,* owner of all in the kingdom).

Joseph was boastful, and God gave him something to boast about.

Moses said he was not a good communicator, and he wrote the first of God's books.

David sinned mightily against God, and God called him "a man after God's own heart."

Jonah ran from God, and God used him to turn others to God.

Elijah was on the verge of suicide, and God used him to raise the dead.

John was a 'son of thunder', but God transformed him into the apostle of love.

Paul persecuted and killed people, and God used him to encourage and give life to many.

In spite of our foibles, God is fabulous!

More Examples of Jesus

As in America today, Isaiah 59:15–21 tells us that truth was failing and that the Lord was looking for people who would intercede for what was going on in the world. The prophet Isaiah and the apostle Paul both mention that believers ought to wear armor so they can pray effectively and always.[9]

Twice, the Gospel records that Jesus wept for others. The most remembered incident was at the death of His good friend, Lazarus. The story contains the shortest verse in the Bible, so many youngsters are quick to memorize the "Jesus wept" line in John 11:35. The second instance of Jesus weeping occurred during His triumphal entry into Jerusalem. "And when He was come near, He beheld the city, and wept over it."[10] Jesus praying, or interceding, for us is further explained in John 17:20, Romans 8:34, and Hebrews 7:25. We must follow His example, especially when dealing with those who are lost in sin.

The Arbitrator that Job longed for is, in reality, Jesus, Who "lay[s] His Hand upon us both" [God and the one praying].[11] Luke 22:32 describes Jesus praying for one of His disciples, while John 17:9 lets us know that Jesus prayed for all of His disciples. He doesn't stop His prayers there; Jesus even prays for all of us who, throughout history, will believe in Him.

Jesus started His risen life by comforting one person, opening up the Scripture to two people, helping the business enterprise of some, feeding others breakfast, restoring one person, and as if foretelling His eternal ministry, Jesus concluded His stay on Earth by blessing those fortunate enough to be in attendance at Bethany when He ascended into the air on that historic day.[12]

Jesus continues His post–earth life by being concerned about your comfort, your business, your cares, your restoration, your understanding of Scripture, your family, and your well-being. Remember that Bethany was the community where Martha was from, and she issued the proclamation that God would give to Jesus anything that He asked.[13] So what did Jesus ask for when He concluded His first earthly visit here? Nothing less than blessings for His people! And Jesus continues requesting such blessings to this very day.[14]

John 12:50 tells us that Jesus speaks whatever the Father says to Him. Because Jesus requested blessings for His followers, we know that the Father is directing Jesus to petition blessings for His children! What tremendous insight into the mind of God! Words cannot express this joy! I am confident that God perpetually honors His Word and wants to give the blessings to us that Jesus requested and continues to request. Jesus ascended into heaven to intercede for you and me. We should ascend to our knees to intercede for all lost souls.

May we not be like the disciples who did not believe the report of Jesus' resurrection. May we believe that Jesus is at the right hand of the God of the universe and eternity. May we believe that He is constantly praying for us. Truly, Jesus is the One who initiated and perpetuates the expression, "God bless you!"

Jesus ascended to intercede, and we ought to do the same.

If this is God's heart, we must emulate His desire and pray, intercede, and plead for those who are lost in the sin of homosexuality. This will remain the right way even as the earth recoils at the rebellion of mankind. As the storms of the Lord come upon earth, the Lord will carry those of us who have His love in our hearts and in our lives. God is carrying us—as the famous poem *Footprints in the Sand* and Psalm 77:19 states—"even when your footprints may not be seen."

8

Out of the Closet and into the Light!

There are those who say that homosexuality is a part of who they are, a part of their DNA. Like so many other things, we are all born with certain predispositions. Some of those predispositions are not good and need to be avoided. Homosexuality is one such behavior.

Homosexuality is no more supposed to remain a part of a person than the desire to covet, lie, cheat, abuse substances, murder, or steal. Colossians 3:5 tells us to *mortify* (kill off, put to death) these things. Other elements of some people's minds, such as depression, personality disorders, suicidal tendencies, and learning disabilities should likewise be evaluated and dealt with appropriately.

As mentioned in the introduction, the same God who instituted the universal laws that society must live by also said homosexuality was forbidden. We can't pick and choose which of His universal laws we will live by. Even if we had the authority to disregard certain laws, humans are cursed with imperfection—how could we ever be certain that the laws we selected to disregard were not the primary ones we needed to obey?

From my personal family experience, I know that there are some people who are naturally prone to certain addictions. Other people are able to disregard these impulses, even after some experimentation. Should we allow those that are more susceptible to such addictions to destroy themselves? Shouldn't we provide some assistance or alert them to possible avenues of escape? There are various resources available to help those who have homosexual leanings, not the least of which is the local church.

A True Story

Here is the true story of someone who was a homosexual and left that lifestyle. For more than twenty years, until 1993, Joseph[1] was involved in the gay scene. More specifically, he was involved in gay ghetto life. This lifestyle was all he had ever known. As a young child, Joseph was sexually abused and lost his father through death. As a young child, he was not able to deal with the trauma of not having a father to protect him, and that trauma was compounded by the sexual abuse.

He was so traumatized, hurt, wounded, disgraced, ashamed, and embarrassed by that abuse, yet the abuse was the very thing that drove him to homosexual behavior. At a very young age, Joseph was addicted to drugs and homosexuality. At the same time, he was trying to forget the pain. He had been shattered, his self-esteem was broken.

The gay ghetto life is characterized by drugs, alcohol, sexual promiscuity, and bars. The resulting violence, crime, hatred, jealousy, and disease became a daily part of his life. Joseph heard television preachers say that God hated gays, and that was a bad blow to him. He felt he had nowhere to go, no one to turn to. And then, one day, an article was delivered to his house entitled "Homosexuality and AIDS." It was written by a famous national television preacher.

Joseph read the article and fell to his knees. He prayed, "God, this is all I have ever known. If you want me to change, you must help me. I cannot do it by myself." A few days later, he left his job and made a commitment to leave the gay lifestyle. Although Joseph knew places to go for drug and alcohol treatment, he didn't know where to go to get help for his gay lifestyle.

Shortly thereafter, he watched an episode of the Phil Donahue Show on television. The episode featured ex-gays who came out of that lifestyle through Jesus Christ. Joseph wrote down the phone number and called immediately. Soon, he received a letter that referred him to a ministry in his hometown. Joseph started attending Emmanuel Ministry every Tuesday night, and he made a few friends. He began to read a book entitled *The LORD Set Me Free.*

He read that book every day, writing down the mentioned verses and studying them in addition to praying. Thus began Joseph's journey toward healing. As he was beginning to grow in his new lifestyle, he knew he needed to attend a church (an idea his support group gave him). Soon, he met up with a friend who was set to attend a revival meeting. Joseph had no idea what a revival was, but when his friend told him it was like church, Joseph asked whether he could go with him. The friend happily obliged.

His friend picked up Joseph in an old car, and they went to the revival meeting. Along the way, Joseph kept telling himself that he was making a big mistake! He wanted to jump out of the car and run to the bars so he could resume the lifestyle that he had known most of his life. They finally made it to the church. It was a small church, and the meeting was held outdoors.

Music was playing when they arrived, and people were sitting in folding chairs. It was the first time in years that Joseph had attended church, and his self-esteem remained shattered. Joseph, scared and insecure, was seated at the front, in the second row, with his friend. He held on by faith while singing, clapping his hands, and doing everything everyone else did. The band that played that night was really great as they praised the Lord.

Afterward, the preacher got up and preached the very things that Joseph was thinking about. It was like a mind reading lecture. Afterward, people were invited to come forward and accept Jesus Christ as Lord and Savior. Eventually, Joseph walked to the front and began to repeat the prayer that was offered for him and all the others who came forward.

An amazing vision entered Joseph's mind when he opened his eyes. He saw Jesus dying. Jesus' life was coming out of Him from the feet and mouth. At the same time, Joseph's sins were coming out of his own feet and mouth and tears. Even though the ground at Calvary was the most horrible ground that Joseph had ever seen, Jesus was the most beautiful being he had ever seen in his life. There was a great love, so great that it melted Joseph.

He cried ugly cries, but at the same time, his tears were beautiful. His Savior, Jesus Christ, was dying. It was so beautiful, and Joseph was at peace. When his friend came by and touched him on his back, Jesus and the scene of Calvary started to disappear. Joseph begged for them not to leave, but to no avail: the vision was gone.

Joseph has never been the same since. His search began because he wanted to know whether God hated him. That memorable night, he learned that our heavenly Father loves us so much that He gave His only Son to die for us. We are loved so much more than anyone can ever imagine. Joseph loves to share that message with anyone who cares to listen. It was the most beautiful vision and life experience Joseph ever had.

Forever changed, he knows he is still not perfect or whole. But he is being transformed by the Holy Spirit each day. Every day, he continues to learn about the Father's love for the brokenhearted. As Joseph puts it, "The truth is, I had to become convicted of the Holy Spirit. I was full of sin, living a lifestyle of sin. And then I had to sincerely repent. I was so lost, I had no idea where to go. I had to fall on my knees and ask for help. And then I had to get up by faith, start searching, start asking, and start praying. And then the Holy Spirit came into my life and showed me that Our Father does not hate me; He loves me. He showed me, showed all of us, His great love for us. After that, it was a big relief. I had finally gotten my answer: He loves me; He loves us. I am not the same person I was before. I have a new life in Jesus Christ, with the Body of Christ, and I have been blessed ever since."

Remember that Joseph's conversion and recovery story began in 1993, a full twenty years from the time of this writing. He remains strong and committed to this day, continuously sharing his life story with others. The new life that he found can be experienced by anyone who chooses Jesus Christ. Joseph continues this new life with the help of another organization that he joined several years ago: Homosexuals Anonymous (HA). With branches worldwide, it is available for anyone seeking freedom from homosexuality. HA assists and encourages gay people to be forthright with their sin and reach out to God for forgiveness and a change of lifestyle. Other homosexuals have far different histories, but the call remains the same:

out of the closet … and into the glorious light! "And God hath both raised up the Lord, and will also raise up us by His Own Power."[2]

God Is Just and Merciful

God is not only just, He is also merciful. God provided a beautiful home for Adam and Eve in the Garden of Eden, and He gave full reign to them with one notable exception. The Lord essentially gave them one commandment to obey, which is exactly what they did not do. Adam and Eve disobeyed God, so they were removed from their beautiful home. After their removal, God was compelled by His own nature to provide a way back for mankind; and that's just what He did.[3] In the same way, God still provides ways out of sinful lifestyles and into glorious living. Indeed, God is merciful.

God still provides ways out of sinful lifestyles and into glorious living!

If we want to be partakers of the divine nature and escape the corruption that is in the world, we must have faith.[4] One of the most quoted Old Testament verses in the New Testament is as follows: "The just shall live by faith."[5] Our spiritual ancestors were commended for their faith

(Hebrews 11). We should walk by faith and not by sight.[6] In other words, we must live by the inner senses of our spirits (i.e., via conscience, intuition, and communion with God), not by our outer senses (e.g., sight and hearing), nor even by the faculties of our soul: mind, will, or emotions. We are to be led by the Spirit of God in our spirits, and then we know that we are the children of God.[7] Faith starts by hearing the Word of God. "Faith comes by hearing and hearing by the Word of God."[8] Jesus told us, "Man shall not live by bread alone, but by every Word that proceeds out of the mouth of God."[9]

The Bible is our faith milk when we are young, and it is our bread and meat when we mature.[10] Follow the Bible and you will be walking in faith. Follow faith and you will be walking by the Word of God.

It Takes Faith

This is a list of what we could not experience without faith:

> Without faith, we would not have peace with God
> (Romans 5:1–2);
> without faith, we could not be saved (Ephesians
> 2:8, 9; 2 Timothy 3:15; Romans 4:16–17);

without faith, we would not be the children of
God (Galatians 3:26);

without faith, we sin (Romans 14:23);

without faith, we would not be purified
(Acts 15:9);

without faith, we would not be justified (Galatians
2:16; 3:8, 24; Romans 3:26, 28, 30);

without faith, we would not be sanctified
(Acts 26:18);

without faith, we would not experience the
righteousness of God (Philippians 3:9;
Galatians 5:5; Romans 3:22; 9:31–32);

without faith, we would not receive the promise
of the Spirit (Galatians 3:14, 22);

without faith, we would not be blessed
(Galatians 3:9);

without faith, we would not have a shield of
protection (Ephesians 6:16; 1 Thessalonians
5:8);

without faith, we would not have a spiritual
foundation (Hebrews 6:1, 2; Acts 20:21);

without faith, we would not be able to stand
spiritually (2 Corinthians 1:24; Romans 5:2;
11:20);

without faith, we would not be kept by the power
of God until the last days (1 Peter 1:5);

without faith, we could not please God
    (Hebrews 11:6);
without faith, our works would be useless
    (James 2:14–26);
without faith, we could not overcome the world
    (1 John 5:4);
without faith, we will not inherit the promises of
    God (Hebrews 4:1–3; 6:12).

(I recommend that all readers of this book speak out loud what we *do* have with faith (e.g., say, "By faith, I have peace with God; by faith, I am saved; with faith, I am blessed; through faith, I will inherit the promises of God.")

All this is in the Bible. Without the Word of God, we could not have faith because "Faith comes by hearing and hearing by the Word of God."[11] Thus, faith enters into us via the Word of God, or it leads us to faith. And because "the just live by faith,"[5] the Word of God is what guides us in our walk of faith. So if we want to be partakers of the divine nature and escape the corruption and lust in the world, we must experience the first in the list of requirements: faith.[12]

Lust refers to many things, but in this case, I am referring to the abnormal sexual lust that a man has for other men, or that a woman has for other women. (Of course, any other sort of lust is also wrong.) Don't ever stop believing that God can change things and make the most out of you. All it takes is a willing heart and a changed attitude. A quote that has guided me for much of my adult life is as follows: "Change comes in the wake of people who face the implications of their own convictions and act upon them."[13] I discovered this phrase on a poster in 1992, and I realized that this philosophy (always looking to become better) encapsulated what I had been striving toward for several years. I sought to live better in every aspect of my life: my family life, my school life, my work life, my financial life, my leisure life, my habits, etc. Such a sentiment can help those who are trapped in the homosexual lifestyle.

The way out can be found in God's Holy Word, the Bible.

Joseph found the way out by experiencing God's Holy Word, which was made real to him. Afterward he encountered several groups that sought to remove the sin of homosexuality from people and bathe them in the glorious light of the Gospel of Jesus Christ. When Joseph thought that his transformation was impossible, he discovered the God of "I'm possible!"

Christians ought to rise up and illustrate the love, concern, and salvation of God to homosexuals and the whole LGBT (lesbian, gay, bisexual, transgender) community. Some are beginning to speak out about their deliverance from this sinful lifestyle, even in the face of America's rush into sin.

Mark Sevillano, Jr. wrote a fantastic book relating his deliverance (due to be released in early 2014). *The Choice I Made When I was Twenty-Three* will impact the multitudes who find it in their search for truth, help, and hope in this area. Some well-known people have experienced freedom from homosexuality, including Dennis Jernigan, Joe Dallas, and Alan Manning Chambers. "It is for freedom that Christ has set us free."[14]

Appendix

This appendix was written as an addition to Chapter One to better understand God's nature, along with mankind's nature, and to indicate some of the similarities and differences. It contains every appropriate instance in the Bible of the phrase "I am", beginning with the references to God's characteristics and ending with mankind's.

The I Am's of God: *I am…*

GOD

Gen. 17:1   the Almighty God
Gen. 26:24   the God of Abraham thy father
Gen. 28:13   the Lord God of Abraham thy father, and
              the God of Isaac
Gen. 31:13   the God of Bethel
Gen. 35:11   God Almighty
Gen. 46:3   God, the God of thy father

Exod. 3:6; Acts 7:32   the God of thy father, the God of Abraham, the God of Isaac, and the God of Jacob

Exod. 3:14   THAT I AM and "…hath sent me unto you."

Exod. 6:2 plus 9 other times in Exodus Lev. 18:5 plus 18 other times in Leviticus; Numbers 3:13,41,45; 1 Kings 20:13, 28; Isaiah 42:8 plus 8 other times in Isaiah; Jeremiah 24:7; 32:27; Ezek. 6:7 plus 55 other times in Ezekiel; Mal. 3:6 the Lord

Exod. 6:7 plus 21 other times in Exodus; Numbers 10:10; Duet. 29:6; Judges 6:10; Isaiah 43:3; 48:17; 51:15; Jer. 9:24; Ezek. 20:5,7,19,20; 28:26; 39:22; Hosea 12:9; 13:4; Joel 2:27; 3:17; Zechariah 10:6 the Lord your {their} God

Exod. 8:22; Joel 2:27   the Lord in the midst of the earth {of Israel}

Exod. 20:5; Deut. 5:9 a jealous God

Exod. 31:13; Lev. 20:8; 22:32; Ezek. 20:12   the Lord that do {which} sanctify {hallow} you

Lev. 20:24,26   the Lord your God {am holy}, which have separated you from other people

Deut. 32:39   He, and there is no god with me

Psalm 46:10; 50:7; Isaiah 43:12; Hosea 11:9 God {even thy God} {and not man}

Isaiah 41:10; Ezek. 34:31   your God

Isaiah 42:8   the Lord: that is My Name

Isaiah 43:3,15; Ezek. 20:5,7,19,20; 39:7; Hosea 13:4 the
Lord your God, the {your} Holy One of
Israel, your Saviour

Isaiah 45:3   the God of Israel

Isaiah 45:5,6,18,22; 46:9   the Lord {God}, and there is
none else {like Me}

Jeremiah 32:27   the Lord, the God of all flesh

Ezek. 13:9; 23:49; 24:24; 28:24; 29:16   the Lord God

Joel 3:17   the Lord your God dwelling in Zion

Matt. 22:32; Mark 12:26 the God of Abraham, Isaac,
and Jacob

Matt. 27:43; John 10:36   the Son of God

Mark 14:62; Luke 22:70   { } [in answer to "Are you the
Christ, the Son of the Blessed {the Son
of God}?"]

John 4:26   I that speak unto thee am He

John 8:24,28; 13:19; 18:5,6,8; Deut. 32:39; Isaiah 41:4;
43:10,13; 46:4; 48:12; 51:12; 52:6   He

Descriptives of God

Gen. 15:1   thy shield, and thy exceeding great reward

Gen. 15:7   the Lord that brought thee out

Exod. 15:26   the Lord that heals you

Exod. 20:2; Lev. 11:45; 19:36; 25:38; 26:13; Numbers 15:41; Deut. 5:6; Psalm 81:10 the Lord your God, which have brought you out of the land of Egypt {to give you the land of Canaan, and to be your God}

Exod. 22:27 gracious (compassionate)

Lev. 11:44,45; 19:2; 20:26; 21:8 holy

Num. 18:20; 44:28 your part and your inheritance

Psalm 35:3 thy salvation

Isaiah 10:13 prudent

Isaiah 43:5 He that blots out your sins

Isaiah 44:24 the Lord that maketh all things

Isaiah 48:17 the Lord thy God which teaches you to profit, which leads you by the way that you should go

Isaiah 49:26; 60:16 your Saviour and your Redeemer

Isaiah 51:12 He that comforts you

Isaiah 52:6 He that does speak

Jeremiah 3:12 merciful

Jeremiah 9:24 the Lord which exercise lovingkindness, judgment, and righteousness, in the earth

Jeremiah 29:23 a witness

Jeremiah 31:9 a Father to Israel

Ezek. 7:9 the Lord that smites

Ezek. 12:11 your sign

Ezek. 20:12 the Lord that sanctify them

Ezek. 44:28	their possession
Zech. 10:6	the Lord their God, and will hear them
Mal. 1:14	a great King
Mal. 3:6	the Lord, I change not
Matt. 11:29	meek and lowly in heart
Matt. 20:15	good
John 6:35, 48	the {that} bread of life
John 6:41,51	the {living} bread which came down from heaven
John 8:12; 9:5; 12:46	the light of the world
John 8:58	Before Abraham was…
John 10:7,9	the door of the sheep
John 10:11,14	the good Shepherd
John 11:25	the resurrection, and the life
John 13:13	Master and Lord…
John 14:6	the way, the truth, and the life
John 15:5,1	the {true} vine
John 17:37	a king
John 19:21	King of the Jews
Acts 9:5; 22:8; 26:15	Jesus whom you persecute
1 Pet. 1:16; Lev. 11:44,45	holy
Rev. 1:18	He that liveth, and was dead; and, behold, I am alive for evermore
Rev. 2:23	He which searches the minds and hearts

Rev. 21:6; 1:8, 11, 17; 22:13; Isaiah 44:6; 48:12 Alpha and Omega, the beginning and the end{ing} {the first and the last}

Rev. 22:16   the root and the offspring of David, and the bright and morning star

Other

Exod. 3:8   come down to deliver them

Deut. 1:42   not among you

2 Kings 21:12   bringing such disaster upon

Isaiah 1:11   full of the burnt offerings

Isaiah 1:14   weary to bear them

Isaiah 41:10   with you: be not dismayed

Isaiah 65:1   sought

Isaiah 65:1   found

Jer. 1:8,19; 15:20; 42:11   with you to deliver you

Jer. 3:14   married unto you

Jer. 15:6   weary with repenting

Jer. 15:20; 30:11; 42:11 with you to save you and to deliver you

Jer. 21:13; 51:25; Ezek. 5:8; 13:8; 21:3; 26:3; 28:22; 29:3,10; 35:3; Nahum 2:13; 3:5   against you

Jer. 23:30,31   against the prophets that steal My Words

Jer. 23:32   against them that prophesy false dreams

Ezek. 13:20   against your magic

Ezek. 16:63   pacified toward you

Ezek. 22:26   profaned among them

Ezek. 30:22   against Pharaoh

Ezek. 34:10   against the shepherds

Ezek. 34:30   with them

Ezek. 36:9   for you

Hosea 14:8   like a green fir tree

Joel 2:27   in the midst of Israel

Haggai 1:13; 2:4   with you {always} {and will bless you} {and will keep you in all places}

Zech. 1:14; 8:2   jealous for Jerusalem and for Zion

Zech. 1:15   very sore displeased with the heathen that are at ease

Zech. 1:16   returned to Jerusalem with mercies

Zech. 8:3   returned unto Zion

Matt. 3:17; 17:5; Mark 1:11; Luke 3:22; 2 Pet. 1:17 well pleased

Matt. 5:17   not come to destroy, but to fulfill

Matt. 9:13   not come to call the righteous, but sinners to repentance

Matt. 9:28   able to do this

Matt. 10:34,35; Luke 12:51   not come to send peace on earth

Matt. 26:32; Mark 14:28   risen {again}

Matt. 28:20; John 13:33; Acts 18:10; Gen. 26:24; 28:15;
Isaiah 41:10; 43:5; Jer. 1:8,19; 15:20;
30:11; 42:11; 46:28; Haggai 1:13; 2:4;
Matt. 28:20   with you

Luke 12:49   come to send fire on the earth

Luke 22:27   among you as He that serves

John 5:43   come in My Father's Name

John 7:28   not come of Myself

John 7:29   from Him

John 8:16; 16:32   not alone

John 8:18   one that bear witness of Myself

John 8:23; 17:16   from above AND not of this {the} world

John 9:5   in the world

John 9:39   come into this world

John 10:10   come that they might have life, and... more abundantly

John 11:15   glad for your sakes

John 12:46   come a light into the world

John 14:10,11,20   in the {My} Father

John 17:10   glorified in them

John 17:11   no more in the world

John 20:17   not yet ascended unto My Father

The I Am's of man: *I am…*

Mortal

Gen. 18:12; 27:2   waxed old

Gen. 25:30   faint

Gen. 25:32   at the point to die

Gen. 27:46   weary of my life

Gen. 49:29   to be gathered unto my people

Deut. 31:2   an hundred and twenty years old this day

Joshua 14:10   this day eighty-five years old

Joshua 23:2   old and stricken in age

Joshua 23:14   going the way of all the earth

Ruth 1:12   too old to have an husband

1 Sam. 12:2; Psalm 71:18   old and grayheaded

2 Sam. 19:35   this day eighty years old

1 Kings 13:31   dead

Job 19:10   gone

Job 30:19   become like dust and ashes

Job 33:6   formed out of the clay

Psalm 6:2; 2 Cor. 11:29; Joel 3:10   weak

Psalm 22:6   a worm

Psalm 22:14   poured out like water

Psalm 31:22; Lam. 3:54   cut off from before Your Eyes

Psalm 38:8   feeble and sore broken

Psalm 88:15   afflicted and ready to die

Psalm 102:11   withered like grass

Psalm 109:23   gone like the shadow

Isaiah 33:24   sick

Isaiah 38:10   deprived of the residue of my years

Lam. 1:14   not able to rise up

Lam. 3:54   cut off

2 Tim. 4;6   now ready to be offered

Descriptives of mankind

Gen. 23:4; Psalm 39:12   a stranger and a sojourner with you

Gen. 24:24   the daughter of

Gen. 24:34   Abraham's servant

Gen. 27:11   a smooth man

Gen. 27:19   Esau thy firstborn

Gen. 32:10   become two bands

Gen. 41:44   Pharaoh

Gen. 45:3,4   Joseph

Joshua 17:14   a great people

Judges 6:15   the least in my father's house

Judges 9:2   your bone and your flesh

Judges 17:9   a Levite

Judges 18:4   his priest

Ruth 2:10   a stranger

Ruth 3:9	Ruth thine handmaid
Ruth 3:12	your near kinsman
1 Sam. 1:15	a woman of a sorrowful spirit
1 Sam. 1:26	the woman that stood by you here, praying unto the Lord
1 Sam. 4:16	he that came out of the army
1 Sam. 9:19	the seer
1 Sam. 17:58	the son of your servant Jesse
1 Sam. 18:23	a poor man, and lightly esteemed
1 Sam. 30:13	a young man
2 Sam. 1:8	an Amalekite
2 Sam. 1:13	the son of a stranger
2 Sam. 14:5	indeed a widow
2 Sam. 19:22	this day king over Israel
2 Sam. 20:17	he
2 Sam. 20:19	one of them that are peaceable and faithful
1 Kings 3:7	but a little child
1 Kings 13:18	a prophet also
1 Kings 18:36; 2 Kings 16:7; Psalm 116:16; 119:125; 143:12	your servant
Job 19:15	an alien in their sight
Job 30:9	their byword
Job 32:6	young
Psalm 119:19	a stranger in the earth
Psalm 119:63	a companion of all them that fear You
Psalm 119:94	Yours

Song of Sol. 2:16; 6:3; 7:10   His {my beloved's}

Isaiah 6:5   undone

Isaiah 6:5   a man of unclean lips

Isaiah 19:11   the son of the wise

Isaiah 44:5   the Lord's

Isaiah 47:8,10   and none else beside me

Jeremiah 1:6   a child

Jeremiah 23:9   a drunken man

Lam. 3:1   the man that has seen affliction by the rod
                  of His Wrath

Ezek. 28:2,9   a god

Jonah 1:9   an Hebrew

Zeph. 2:15   and there is none beside me

Zech. 13:5   no prophet

Zech. 13:5   a farmer

Matt. 8:9; Luke 7:8   a man under authority

Matt. 24:5; Mark 13:6; Luke 21:8   Christ

Luke 5:8; 18:13   a sinful man

Luke 18:11   not as other men are

John 1:20; 3:28; Acts 13:25   not the Christ

John 1:23   the voice of one crying in the wilderness

Acts 10:21   he whom ye seek

Acts 21:39; 22:3   a man

Acts 23:6   a Pharisee

Acts 27:23   God's

Rom. 1:14   debtor

Rom. 7:14   carnal, sold under sin

Rom. 7:24   a wretched man!

Rom. 11:1   an Israelite

Rom. 11:13   the apostle of the Gentiles

1 Cor. 13:2   nothing

1 Cor. 15:9   the least of the apostles

2 Cor. 12:10; 11:29   weak, then am I strong

Eph. 3:8   less than the least of all saints

Eph. 6:20   an ambassador in bonds

1 Tim. 1:15   chief sinner

1 Peter 5:1   also an elder, a witness of the sufferings of
                Christ, and a partaker of the glory

Weaknesses of mankind

Gen. 43:14   bereaved

Exod. 4:10   not eloquent

Exod. 4:10   slow of speech

Exod. 6:12,30   of uncircumcised lips

Num. 11:14; Deut. 1:9   not able to bear all this people
                alone

Judges 4:19   thirsty

1 Sam. 28:15; Lam. 1:20   sore distressed

2 Sam. 1:26   distressed for you

2 Sam. 3:39   this day weak, though anointed king

2 Sam. 24:14; 1 Chron. 21:13   in a great strait

1 Kings 14:6   sent to you with heavy tidings

1 Kings 22:34; 2 Chron. 18:33; 35:23   wounded {sore}

Ezra 9:6   ashamed and blush to lift up my face

Job 7:4   full of tossings to and fro

Job 7:8   not

Job 7:20   a burden to myself

Job 9:28   afraid of all my sorrows

Job 10:15   full of confusion

Job 12:4   as one mocked of his neighbor

Job 19:7   not heard

Job 19:20   escaped with the skin of my teeth

Job 21:6; Psalm 56:3; Jer. 38:19   afraid

Job 23:15   afraid of Him

Job 40:5   vile (unworthy)

Psalm 6:6   weary with my groaning

Psalm 25:16   desolate and afflicted

Psalm 28:7   helped

Psalm 31:9; 69:17; 102:2   in trouble

Psalm 31:12   forgotten

Psalm 31:12   like a broken vessel

Psalm 38:6   troubled

Psalm 38:6   bowed down greatly

Psalm 39:10   consumed by the blow of Thine Hand

Psalm 40:12   not able to look up

Psalm 40:17; 70:5; 86:1; 109:22   poor and needy

Psalm 69:2   come into deep waters

Psalm 69:3   weary of my crying

Psalm 69:8   become a stranger unto my brethren

Psalm 69:20   full of heaviness

Psalm 69:29   poor and sorrowful

Psalm 71:7   as a wonder unto many

Psalm 77:4   so troubled

Psalm 88:4   counted with them that go down into the pit

Psalm 88:4   as a man that has no strength

Psalm 88:8   confined

Psalm 88:15   distracted

Psalm 109:23   tossed up and down

Psalm 119:107   afflicted very much

Psalm 119:120   afraid of Your Judgments

Psalm 119:141; Lam. 1:11   small and despised

Psalm 142:6   brought very low

Prov. 30:2   more ignorant than any man

Isaiah 21:8   set in my ward whole nights

Isaiah 29:12   not learned

Isaiah 38:14   oppressed

Isaiah 65:5   holier than you

Jeremiah 2:23   not polluted

Jeremiah 4:19   pained at my very heart

Jeremiah 6:11   weary with holding in

Jeremiah 8:21   dismayed

Jeremiah 20:7   in derision daily

Jeremiah 36:5   shut up

Lam. 1:11   despised

Lam. 1:20   in distress

Hosea 12:8; Zech. 11:5   become rich

Jonah 2:4   cast out of Thy Sight

Habak. 2:1   reproved

Zech. 11:5; Hosea 12:8   rich

Matt. 3:11; 8:8; Mark 1:7; Luke 3:16; 7:6; 15:19,21; John 1:27; Acts 13:25; Gen. 32:10; Job 40:4   not worthy

Matt. 27:24   innocent of the blood of this man

Luke 16:3   ashamed

Luke 16:4   put out

Luke 16:24   tormented

Luke 22:58; John 18:17,25,27   not

Rom. 11:3; 1 Kings 19:10,14   only left

Acts 26:2,7   accused

Acts 28:20   bound

2 Peter 1:13   in this tabernacle

Other

Exod. 3:19   sure

Lev. 8:35; 10:13   commanded

Num. 22:38   come unto you

Deut. 26:3   come unto the country which the Lord sware unto our fathers for to give us

Joshua 14:11   as strong this day

Judges 8:5	pursuing after
Judges 19:18	now going to the house of the Lord
Ruth 4:4	after you
1 Sam. 14:7	with you according to your heart
1 Sam. 16:2,5	come to sacrifice unto the Lord
2 Sam. 11:5	with child
2 Sam. 14:15	come to speak of this thing
2 Sam. 19:20	come the first this day
1 Kings 8:20; 2 Chron. 6:10	risen up in the room of David my father
1 Kings 19:4	not better than my fathers
1 Kings 19:10,14	only left
2 Chron. 2:9	about to build shall be wonderful great
Neh. 6:3	doing a great work
Job 10:7	not wicked
Job 11:4	clean in your eyes
Job 12:3; 13:2	not inferior to you
Job 32:18	full of matter
Job 33:6	according to thy wish in God's stead
Job 33:9	clean without transgression
Job 33:9; Jer. 2:35	innocent
Job 34:5	righteous
Psalm 13:4	moved
Psalm 17:3	purposed that my mouth shall not sin
Psalm 22:2	not silent
Psalm 52:8	like a green olive tree in the house of God

Psalm 73:23; Psalm 139:18   continually {still} with you

Psalm 86:2   holy

Psalm 120:7   for peace

Psalm 139:14   fearfully and wonderfully made

Eccles. 1:16   come to great estate

Isaiah 44:16   warm

Jeremiah 6:11   full of the fury of the Lord

Jeremiah 15:16   called by Your Name

Jeremiah 26:14   in your hand

Ezek. 27:3   of perfect beauty

Micah 3:8   full of power by the Spirit of the Lord

Micah 7:1   as when they have gathered the summer fruits

Luke 16:4   resolved

Luke 22:33   ready to go with Thee

Acts 9:10   here

Acts 18:6   clean

Acts 20:26   pure from the blood of all men

Acts 21:13; 2 Tim. 4:6   ready not to be bound only, but also to die at Jerusalem for the name of the Lord Jesus

Acts 26:25   not mad

Acts 26:26; Romans 8:38; 14:14; 15:14; 2 Tim. 1:5,12   persuaded

Rom. 1:15   ready to preach the gospel

Rom. 1:16; 2 Tim. 1:12   not ashamed of the gospel of Christ

Rom. 15:29   sure

Rom. 16:19   glad therefore on your behalf

1 Cor. 1:12; 3:4   of Paul

1 Cor. 3:4   of Apollos

1 Cor. 9:2   to you [an apostle]

1 Cor. 9:22   made all things to all men

1 Cor. 11:1   of Christ

1 Cor. 13:12   known

1 Cor. 15:10   what I am [by the grace of God]

1 Cor. 16:17   glad

2 Cor. 7:4   filled with comfort

2 Cor. 7:4   exceeding joyful in all our tribulation

2 Cor. 7:14   not ashamed

2 Cor. 11:2   jealous over you with Godly jealousy

2 Cor. 11:21   bold also

2 Cor. 11:23; Col. 1:23,25   more [a minister]

2 Cor. 12:11   become a fool in glorying

2 Cor. 12:14   ready to come to you

2 Cor. 13:1   coming to you

Gal. 2:20   crucified with Christ

Gal. 4:12; 1 Kings 22:4; 2 Kings 3:7; 2 Chron. 18:3 as you are

Philip. 1:17   set for the defence of the gospel

Philip. 1:23   in a strait between the two

Philip. 3:12	apprehended of Christ Jesus
Philip. 4:11	therewith to be content
Philip. 4:12	instructed
Philip. 4:18	full
Col. 4:3	also in bonds
1 Tim. 2:7; 2 Tim. 1:11	ordained {appointed} a preacher, and an apostle, and a teacher
2 Tim. 1:12	not ashamed

(Although several of these references may be placed in more than one category, I have only listed each once.)

Author's personal NOTES:

I am this or that or the other may not ordinarily speak of humility; however, some Bible verses where this phrase occurs do speak of humility. (1 Cor. 13:2 "...I am nothing"; 15:10 "But by the grace of God I am what I am...; Gal. 2:20 "I am crucified with Christ..."; Eph. 3:7-8 do speak of humility).

Think of the true "I AM" of Exodus 3:6,14. God is not the "I was" or "I will be", He is not for yesterday or tomorrow, He is for your today. He is the same yesterday, today, and forever (Malachi

3:6+) so He is for you today, He can do the same things he did for others in the past and will do for others in the future.

Many times Jesus said, "I am..."

Enter your own personal NOTES from what you see in this appendix:

Chapter Notes

Introduction
[1] 1 Peter 4:8; James 5:20
[2] Isaiah 26:2, 3, 7
[3] Psalm 5:7; 51:1; 69:13, 16; 106:7, 45

Chapter 1
[1] John 3:17; John 12:47, 48
[2] Luke 9:55–56
[3] Exodus 25:21–22a
[4] Francis A. Schaeffer, *No Little People* (Downers Grove: InterVarsity Press, 1974), 112.
[5] John 3:17
[6] Ibid
[7] John 10:10
[8] Colossians 1:29
[9] Psalm 103
[10] James Strong, *Abingdon's Strong's Exhaustive Concordance of the Bible: Dictionary of the Greek Testament* (Nashville: Abingdon, 1890), 77 (#5485).
[11] Genesis 2:7
[12] 2 Timothy 3:16, 17
[13] Ephesians 2:8–10
[14] John 5:39
[15] 1 Corinthians 15:45

Chapter 2
[1] 1 Corinthians 13:7

2 Luke 22:32
3 1 Corinthians 13:8
4 Romans 5:8
5 Luke 9:51–56; 1 John 3:16
6 Matthew 7:21
7 John 12:47, 48
8 D. Elton Trueblood. BrainyQuote.com, Xplore Inc, 2012. *http://www.brainyquote.com/quotes/authors/d/d elton trueblood. html*, (accessed April 24, 2012).
9 Hebrews 11:2
10 Romans, chapters 1–3
11 James 1:22; Romans 2:13; Ephesians 2:10

Chapter 3

1 1 Corinthians 6:9–10
2 1 Corinthians 6:11
3 Genesis 2:18
4 Genesis 1:28
5 Ephesians 5:23
6 Genesis 9:7
7 Isaiah 5:21; Proverbs 5:21-23; Jeremiah 5:21
8 D. Elton Trueblood. BrainyQuote.com, Xplore Inc, 2012. *http://www.brainyquote.com/quotes/authors/d/d eltontrueblood. html*, (accessed April 24, 2012).
9 Isaiah 5:20
10 Psalm 19:11; Romans 6:23; John 1:1–3
11 Leviticus 20:13
12 Isaiah 1:9–17
13 Isaiah 1:17
14 Mark 1:15
15 Hebrews 6:1, 2; Derek Prince, *The Foundation Series: Repent & Believe* (Ft. Lauderdale: Derek Prince Ministries), 9–17.

Chapter 4

1 2 Peter 1:21; 2 Timothy 3:16; Jeremiah 36:4; Acts 28:25
2 Genesis 11:6

[3]   David Wilkerson, *America's Last Call* (Lindale, TX: Wilkerson Trust Publications, 1998), 56.

Chapter 5

[1]   1 John 2:17

[2]   Matthew 24:35; Mark 13:31; Luke 21:33

[3]   Matthew Clark. "Mother Teresa's Defense of the Unborn at the U.S. Supreme Court," July 25, 2012, http://aclj.org/pro-life/mother-teresa-defense-unborn-us-supreme-court, (accessed August 26, 2013).

[4]   Phil Keaggy, (1980). Little Ones. On *Ph'lip Side* [Album]. Brentwood, Tennessee: Sparrow Records, a division of EMI Christian Music Group.

[5]   Proverbs 22:6

[6]   Psalm 127:3

Chapter 6

[1]   *United States v. Windsor,* 570 U.S. ___(2013) (Scalia, A., dissenting), page 5. http://www.supremecourt.gov/opinions/12pdf/12-307_6j37.pdf, (accessed June 30, 2013).

[2]   Ron Crews. "Chaplain endorsers: DOMA decision reinforces need for conscience protection language recently passed by the House of Representatives," June 26, 2013, http://chaplainalliance.org/site/wp-content/uploads/2013/06/2013-06-26-Chaplain-Alliance-News-Release.pdf, (accessed August 26, 2013).

[3]   Genesis 18:24

[4]   Genesis 13:13

[5]   C.S. Lewis, *Mere Christianity*, revised edition (New York: Macmillan/Collier, 1952), 55–56.
      Josh McDowell, Evidence That Demands a Verdict, revised edition (San Bernardino: Here's Life Publishers, 1979), 104.

[6]   "San Antonio Human Rights Coalition," http://sahumanrightscoalition.org, (accessed September 1, 2013).

[7]   George O. Wood, "Statement of George O. Wood, General Superintendent of the Assemblies of God, Regarding United

States Supreme Court Same-Sex Marriage Cases June 26, 2013," http://ag.org/newsletters/official/AGministers/AG_062613/AG.htm, (accessed June 27, 2013).

8   "Court Tells Christians: There's a 'Price' for Your Beliefs," Alliance Defending Freedom, http://www.alliancedefendingfreedom.org/page/Elane-Photography, (accessed August 24, 2013).

9   "Anti-Christian Persecution & Oppression in Canada: The high cost of legalizing same-sex marriage (SSM)," Campaign Life Coalition 2010, http://www.campaignlifecoalition.com/shared/media/editor/file/ Persecution_of_Christians-SSM_revJun28-2013.pdf, (accessed July 9, 2013).

10   1 Kings 14:22–24; 15:11–12; 22:43, 46

11   John 12:47, 48

12   Hebrews 10:24–27

13   Genesis 3:1

14   Mark 12:28

15   Exodus 20:1–17; Deuteronomy 5:6–21

16   John 3:16; 1 John 3:16

Chapter 7

1   John 8:11

2   Ruben Duarte, as told by his wife, September 8, 2013.

3   John 16:8

4   Leviticus 19:18; Matthew 5:43; Matthew 19:19; Matthew 22:39; Mark 12:31; Luke 10:27; Romans 13:9; Galatians 5:14; James 2:8

5   Leviticus 18:22

6   John 8:3–11

7   Genesis 18:25

8   Genesis 18:19

9   Ephesians 6:10–18; Isaiah 59:17

10   Luke 19:41

11   Job 9:32–35

12   Luke 24:50–51

[13] John 11:1, 21–22
[14] Hebrews 7:25; 5:7; Romans 8:34

Chapter 8

[1] Joseph is the assumed name of a real person.
[2] 1 Corinthians 6:14
[3] St. Augustine, *Basic Writings of Saint Augustine: The Enchiridion* (Grand Rapids: Baker Book House, 1992), 673–674.
[4] 2 Peter 1:4–5
[5] Romans 1:17; Galatians 3:11; Hebrews 10:38; Habakkuk 2:4
[6] 2 Corinthians 5:7
[7] Romans 8:14; Watchman Nee, *The Spiritual Man* (New York: Christian Fellowship Publishers, Inc., 1968).
[8] Romans 10:17
[9] Matthew 4:4
[10] 1 Peter 2:2; 1 Corinthians 3:2; Hebrews 5:14
[11] Romans 10:17
[12] 2 Peter 1:4–5
[13] Unknown author.
[14] Galatians 5:1a (NIV)